WHERE'S THE NURSE?

Published by

Librario Publishing Ltd

ISBN: 978-1-904440-76-5

Copies can be ordered via the Internet
www.librario.com

or from:

Brough House, Milton Brodie, Kinloss
Moray IV36 2UA
Tel /Fax No 00 44 (0)1343 850 178

Printed and bound by Biddles Ltd, King's Lynn, Norfolk

Where's The Nurse?

By Margaret Stewart

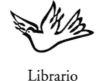

Librario

The Author

Margaret Stewart was born in England and came to live in Glasgow in 1952. She was educated at Whitehill School in Dennistoun. She trained as a general nurse in Glasgow Royal Infirmary, and as a midwife at the Eastern General Hospital. Margaret Stewart worked as a staff nurse in Glasgow both in the Royal and Western Infirmaries. After she was married she moved to Aberdeen and worked as a part time staff nurse in Aberdeen Royal Infirmary. She then qualified as a district nurse and worked as a district nursing sister in Aberdeen. Whilst working on the district, Margaret Stewart developed her knowledge of palliative care, and became a teacher of district nurse students in the practical aspects of their work.

During her nursing life, Margaret Stewart met and recalled many patients, she remembers the good times and the bad, and in this story describes the many changes that have occurred in the nursing profession for better or worse. The patients and nurses are all real people and every incident described is true, only the names have been altered.

Margaret Stewart is a wife, a mother and a grandmother. She lives in Aberdeen and enjoys hill walking and spending time with her five grandchildren.

Chapter 1: The survival of the fittest

Whenever I was asked "What will you do when you leave school?" I only had one answer - I want to be a nurse. My grandmother told me that nursing was hard work. Brought up on a farm in the windswept Orkney islands, Granny knew what she was talking about - but how could I have any idea what she really meant? At eighteen I felt I could conquer the world. I applied to do nurse training, and in May 1960 with some other young hopefuls, all as apprehensive as myself, I was ushered into a classroom in the Glasgow Royal Infirmary.

We chatted nervously. Most of us were local but one girl had come from Perth, a long distance compared with my 15 minute journey on the 102 trolley bus along Royston Road and off at Castle Street right at the hospital door. She had brought an orange for her return journey. It sat on her desk, a bright splash of colour. It cheered me up during the essay writing and dictation tests, following which we were interviewed separately by the matron and a senior tutor.

The name 'matron' conjures up a formidable woman riding the high seas of hospital life like a ship in full sail, but this was a frail little lady in a grey dress and a starched cap. She would retire from the hospital during the next year but, full of presence and dignity, she made each of us feel it was a great honour to be accepted for training in this teaching hospital. After all, Lord Lister had pioneered antiseptic surgery here but the laurels didn't only go to the medical profession. The very first matron had been one of Florence Nightingale's nurses. The lady with the lamp had left a lasting legacy. Her aim had been to train young women to be ladies as well as nurses and her word was still law among the nursing sisters who would teach us the discipline and craft of our profession.

Buoyed up by being told we had passed, we went back into the classroom - and there on the desk was that solitary orange. To this day I can see it sitting there. Its owner had failed the interview, a sobering reminder that difficulties lay ahead to be faced and hopefully conquered.

We were not to be let loose in a hospital until we had completed a three month probationary period in pre-nursing school. This was a separate building in Glasgow's West End, housed within the elegant portals of three Victorian terraced houses. The dedication and demeanour of the Sister Tutors, Miss Black and Miss Clark, were what you could expect in a convent. Miss Black informed us in her opening talk, "The primary function of nurses is service. The nursing profession exists solely to assist and actively support the well-being of mankind. Our tuition will ensure that you learn how to create an atmosphere conducive to the patient's physical, social and spiritual well-being."

After this awe-inspiring preamble we were shown to rooms we would call home for the next three months. We were all strangers, quartered two or three to a room. I shared with Sally and Carol. We chatted as we unpacked. Sally laughed as she ripped open a packet of black nylon stockings. 'Hey, dig these! How's this for style!'

"Yes, and they cost me ten and sixpence," I said. "Ordinary nylons are only three bob a pair. Where did you get yours, girls?"

Those black nylon stockings, such an essential part of our nurse's uniform but not readily available in local shops, had taken us on a foray through the select department stores along Sauchiehall Street: Treron, Copland and Lyle, Pettigrew and Stephen.

"What about these clumpy black shoes? They're just what my mother always says are good for your feet," Carol joked as we tied shoe laces for the first time for years. Our fashion shoes with high heels were consigned to the back of the locker and we turned our attention to the starched caps and collars, aprons, purple and white striped cotton dresses and a navy cloak lined with red all neatly laid out on the bed. This uniform had hardly changed in the last half century.

8

Gales of laughter accompanied our fashion parade: uniforms had been issued with little regard to individual size. Six-foot Aileen appeared at our door and struck a mannequin pose – she had been given a skimpy short dress. Behind her Joan, all of four foot ten, bunched up a dress so long it trailed across the floor. But we sorted ourselves out and when we put on the uniform we felt as though we were on the road to being professional nurses. The cloaks certainly added to our distinctive appearance and we all enjoyed wearing our uniforms, not least when one of our boy friends said "your outfit makes plain girls look pretty, and pretty girls look stunning" - which was not what the sister tutors had in mind at all.

The first hurdle we encountered next morning was making our beds in the correct hospital style before going down to breakfast. We had been warned that the penalty for not meeting the required standard was to be hauled out of the classroom to remake your bed. I can't remember this dire threat being carried out but we lived in fear that it would be, so we tucked the starched sheets under the mattress in a neat triangle known as an envelope corner. Our pillows had to be positioned with the open end of the pillow case facing the wall. We only finally left the room when we'd checked that each cotton bedspread had been smoothed without a crease.

One night, while Sally was asleep her pillow fell out of bed on to an electric night storage heater. "Look at this girls, whatever will I do," she wailed next morning, pointing to the charred remains of her feather pillow with its thick striped twill covering. "What will Miss Black say?"

"Cheer up, Sally, it will give the old dragon something to think about, then she'll not worry if our sheets aren't tucked in right," Carol consoled her.

"Let's stuff it in the bucket and hope it's emptied before she inspects the rooms," I suggested.

We fled down to breakfast, but nothing could be hidden from the eagle eyes of the stern senior sister tutor. We were all sitting in the class when Miss Black marched in. "Look at this," she stormed, holding up the offending object. "You must learn more respect for hospital property!"

After she'd left the room wee Joan remarked, "You could have been burnt in your beds, you three girls, but all she cared about was that lumpy old hospital pillow!"

Most of our time was spent in the classroom where Miss Black and Miss Clark taught principles of nursing. "Who is the most important person in the hospital?" Miss Black asked. "The matron" we chorused. "No of course not, it's the patient, and don't you ever forget that," she answered sternly.

No, we weren't in any danger of forgetting – we just wanted to get there and start caring for real people but first we had to study anatomy and physiology, also Latin abbreviations used in drug prescribing: *b.i.d., bis in die* twice a day; *t.i.d., ter in die*, three times a day, or, confusingly *t.d.s., ter di sumendum*, which also meant three times a day, while *o.n., omne nocte*, meant every evening

We studied nutrition and invalid cookery. This was a light relief from textbooks. We went off to the kitchen and made scrambled egg, steamed whiting and parsley sauce and a variety of milk puddings that we then presented to the tutors for criticism before sampling each other's efforts.

Our health and hygiene course took us outside to look at damp proofing and drains – no, we weren't training to be plumbers. We had to understand the connection between insanitary housing and diseases rampant in Glasgow such as tuberculosis, para-typhoid fever and gastro-enteritis in small babies.

Back inside it was time for a spot of bed making. Bed making practice was done in the classroom without the added worry of having a real patient in the bed: we pretended by taking it in turns to be 'bodies'. None of us had realised that there were so many different ways of doing such a mundane task.

We learnt how to make beds to receive patients on admission to the ward, theatre beds, beds for steam kettles used to treat chest infections, cot beds, and the special technique of arranging sheets and blankets for patients on traction. This word 'traction' was a mystery. Did it have something to do with farms? No, it seemed to be about weights and pulleys, which made me think of the kitchen at home with washing dripping on the wooden pulley after the weekly labour at the sink. In fact traction was for people with broken legs – or as our tutor said, a fractured shaft of femur.

Tray and trolley setting was an essential part of our course. All dressings for wound care were made up, packed and sterilised, then reused. Every practical procedure from bathing patients in bed to complex dressings required bowls, basins, instruments and lotions to be set up on a tray or trolley. We had to remember the correct items for each course of action.

"It's all so complicated isn't it, Margaret?" Carol whispered, and I nodded. "Perhaps it will all make sense when we're actually on the wards," we reassured one another.

So over mince and mashed potatoes at lunch-time we would rehearse, "Trolley for bathing a patient in bed… a long rubber mackintosh to protect the floor and a draw mackintosh to go under the patient, a large basin of water…"

"Yes, but, oh help, what temperature is it?" Sally asked. "I know, it's 105 degrees Fahrenheit… but what about the bath thermometer, which wee metal dish does it go in…"

"It's not a metal dish, it's a gallipot," Carol reminded her, "But where do we put it on the trolley – top shelf or bottom?"

As probationers we were nevertheless salaried employees, paid £9 per month for a forty-two hour week with bed and board provided. The hours spent in classroom corresponded to the shift patterns of the wards: eight a.m. to five p.m. with a split shift on a Wednesday. One Wednesday afternoon Sally, Carol and I went horse riding. The horses seemed very big when we got close. Was this really a good idea? No riding boots or jockey caps for us, but undaunted, we climbed into the saddles and tried to canter off. Carol's horse went under a low branch, leaving her stuck up the tree.

"What's she doing up there?" I wondered but I couldn't stop to find out. My horse decided it was training for the Derby and galloped away with me clinging on to the reins in desperation. Sally meanwhile couldn't get her horse to start.

"Wait for me, I'm being left behind," she called.

Carol got down from her perch, my mount gave up its dreams of fame and fortune and we went back to the stables, breathlessly greeting each other, "Are you all right? Will we come back for another go next week? I'll never get on to a horse again... at least it's made a change from lectures..."

However, by five o'clock we were back in our uniform for four more hours in the classroom, studying the four stages in the life of pulex irritans, the human flea. We learnt how this nasty parasite entered the body and how to get rid of it. We noted that it has hooked feet and very strong back legs for jumping – unlike our horses, we joked afterwards over bedtime drinks – cocoa made with hot water.

"My Mum heaps in three spoons of drinking chocolate and always makes it with milk," I sighed. "And imagine we all have to be tucked up in bed at eleven o'clock!"

"It sure puts a stopper on your social life," Carol said gloomily.

And indeed, I still wonder how we managed to get engaged or married, but by the end of three years some of us had achieved a diamond ring as well as our nursing certificate and hospital badge.

But for now we sat in the classroom in our new uniforms whilst the sister tutors tried to mould us into nurses.

A week in a real hospital ward was the next step. Dressed in full uniform, including those eye-catching cloaks, we were driven across Glasgow in a green and orange double decker Corporation bus.

"Well, girls, this is it at last," we agreed, caught between excitement and apprehension. We teenagers were about to be let loose on unsuspecting patients who thought we were special because we wore purple armbands which in fact only designated our lowly status. Little did those patients realise how nervous we were! I still remember the long line of beds, all so beautifully made with their white starched sheets and counterpanes. It was all exactly to the standard taught in the classroom but the difference was there were real people in those beds who needed to be fed and washed, helped out of bed to sit in a chair – and I was one of the nurses they called for. I was now part of a team who would have to cope with all emergencies. Suppose somebody died? They might even have diarrhoea! The classroom seemed a long way away!

We made beds, gave out bedpans, helped to feed and wash patients, and started to believe we could become 'proper' nurses. Sister, however, was unimpressed if we had forgotten to roll up the rubber mackintosh, or had not laid it neatly on the bottom shelf of the bathing trolley, or if we had left the tin of dusting powder on the locker of a previous patient during our expedition up and down the ward on the bathing round.

My first job was to delouse an old lady's hair. She was lying flat in bed and I tried to remember classroom tuition as I got to work dragging a fine toothed bone comb through straggling grey hair, dabbing on a solution of lorexane from a brown bottle, first making sure I had spread a waterproof cape over the feather pillow.

Then there was the bedpan round! I went to the white-tiled sluice at the top of the ward with another junior nurse. We sprayed stainless steel bedpans with steaming hot water to warm them up for the comfort of the patients. Then down the long ward we trundled the trolley. We lifted helpless patients with paralysed limbs on to warm bedpans, then went back and took them all off again. The other junior nurses seemed to work at a great speed, how would I ever catch up with them? Nowadays, watching the flight attendants pushing the food trolleys up and down an aeroplane, I am reminded of those bedpan trolleys. Thankfully the ones on the planes smell much better!

After the patients' lunch the whole nursing team gathered round the sister, to be given the 'report'. We stood around her wooden desk at the bottom of the ward with our pencils and notepads at the ready to be informed about every patient's care; "Mrs Smith, 2 oz water every hour, Miss Brown may get up to sit for half an hour, Mrs Anderson is to have a barium meal –" whatever's that" I thought – "tomorrow, so she will fast from 12 midnight."

No concessions were made to help beginners understand what was going on. The week in the wards proved to be a make or break experience for some of us; some trainee nurses were already beginning to change their minds about a nursing career.

Back in the college we prepared for our first written tests. Girls in starched caps could be seen wandering up and down the lofty Victorian staircase dreamily reciting "Bowels: a regular daily action is necessary... Tudor Edwards' spectacles are used for giving oxygen...a bowl for the dentures goes at the front right hand-side of the tray for cleaning the mouth... The loop of Henle is in the kidney... the tympanic membrane is situated at the deepest part of the external auditory canal..."

We'd all heard about wiping the fevered brow but basic nursing care involved more than any of us had imagined. I realised that staying the course was going to be the survival of the fittest – but I'd started and I was determined to go on.

Chapter 2: First Impressions

Our new life as student nurses began in the Nurses' Home. Nobody of the male species was allowed through the doors. The austere rooms were on three floors with an old-fashioned lift wheezing up and down.

"They've put us on different floors so it won't be so easy to meet," Carol remarked.

Each room had a bed, a wardrobe, a chest of drawers and a chair. There were no facilities for making tea or coffee. Our uniforms were sent to the hospital laundry and personal washing was done in the bathroom. We soaked ourselves in the bath using unlimited hot water with long strings of other people's undies dripping on top of us. Showers were non-existent – but they were unheard of in most homes in Glasgow at that time.

Everyone had to be in by midnight – if we wanted to stay out later we had to submit a written request to Matron. When we were on duty until 9 p.m. we had to be back in the Home by eleven. To snatch a brief date with a boyfriend we would rush off duty, dab on Max Factor crème puff, add a dash of our favourite scent, trying to disguise the fact we'd spent the last nine hours running up and down the wards non-stop.

Residence in the Home was compulsory for the first two years, even if, like me, you lived within travelling distance of the hospital. Students came from all over Scotland. Many, especially those from the Western Isles, could only go home once a year.

The first morning we assembled in the dining room for breakfast at seven fifteen. Our uniforms looked so new, and we did too, among hundreds of more senior, self-assured girls. We all hoped to be sent to the surgical wards where the excitement of patients "going to theatre" and having wounds dressed or stitches taken out made the work seem glamorous and exciting. Everyone dreaded being sent to a ward with a tyrannical sister. This had happened to Sally during her probationary week on the wards and we spent the next four weeks building up her damaged self-esteem. Was this ordeal in store for me?

The assistant matron came in for Roll Call – the daily procedure took place immediately after breakfast. This superior lady was immaculate in a green dress and a cap with a frill.

She sat in an office all day, attending to mysteriously important affairs. She called out everybody's name. If you failed to answer "Present" everybody knew you had committed the dreadful crime of sleeping in. We sat in total silence while she went through a list of four hundred names. "Nurse So and So… assist Ward Such and Such…"

I was allocated a female medical ward. I have nursed hundreds of people since then, but I can still see these, my first patients, as clearly as when I walked into the ward on that first day. I can visualise the beds they were lying in, their faces and their hair colour.

Miss Smith, a woman in her forties with a fresh complexion had multiple sclerosis. Her glasses slipped down her nose as she lay in bed. She was unable to push them back in place, to stand or walk unaided, or wash and feed herself.

Next to her, Mrs McDonald had congestive cardiac failure. She was nursed sitting up day and night. In the classroom we had learned how to make a cardiac bed. Then it was just a name, now as I pulled out the metal back rest and piled six pillows into an armchair position I saw how this enabled Mrs McDonald to breathe more easily.

Granny Clark had diabetes. (All the old ladies were known as Granny and the old men were Pop, no Christian names were ever used.) Granny Clark wore a purple dressing gown and used to love the attention of the nurses when we cared for her in bed, but she resisted our attempts to get her up to walk. 'Och, hen, I cannae walk the day, I'm no feeling awfu' weel. I'll jist sit here in ma chair and hae a wee rest,' she'd say. She was one of the patients from the tenement flats around the hospital without a bath or hot water: being in hospital was a rest from the difficulties of life.

Another patient I remember well, Mrs Douglas, had had a stroke which paralysed her down her right side and meant that she couldn't speak. I had never met anyone who had lost the power of speech and I felt so inadequate trying to understand her. She was only fifty with nicotine stained fingers, the same nicotine that had furred up her arteries. The association between smoking and arterial thrombosis wasn't understood. Hospital wards were wreathed in a haze of cigarette smoke at the patients' rest hour after lunch, and indeed doctors prescribed tobacco to help people with asthma, as it encouraged them to cough.

Two ladies in adjacent beds had both had heart attacks, and during the six weeks of enforced bed rest they became good friends. Mrs Taylor went home the day before Mrs Brown. Just then, we had a phone call, Mrs Taylor was to be readmitted after another coronary thrombosis. Sister told Mrs Brown the news. While they were still speaking, word came that Mrs Taylor died in the ambulance. Mrs Brown was shocked and so was I. But I was being trained not to show my feelings or become emotionally involved with the patients so I absorbed myself in the work of the ward.

Bedmaking was an important daily ritual. We changed the sheets every day, putting the top sheet to the bottom and giving a fresh top sheet. The patients in the freshly made beds were frightened to breathe in case they spoiled the starched crispness of the sheets.

Soiled bed linen had to be sluiced down by the junior nurse. Sheets, blankets, pillow cases and counterpanes, towels and patients' night-clothes were piled up in heaps on the floor of the sluice, ticked off on a list and packed into a wicker laundry basket. This was also one of the tasks tackled by the most junior nurses.

Syringes, needles, blood transfusion and intravenous infusion sets, catheters, drainage tubes and bottles for the drainage of wounds or urine were all sterilised and re-used. Nothing was disposable, except the harassed nurses!

Who was the most important person in the hospital? The patient seemed to come far down the list when cleaning and scrubbing took so much time. There was so much to do that sometimes you felt you couldn't cope with the cry, "Nurse" from somebody in the ward. When I saw my friends in the dining room, I never let on if things were getting me down, and neither did they, instead we talked 'shop' and swapped stories about our patients.

Sally worked in a male surgical ward. "This man came in bleeding all over the place. Imagine, he'd tried to kill himself. He'd swallowed broken glass. They poured loads of blood into him before he went to theatre."

It made my medical ward seem very tame!

"Well, we had a lady admitted who must weigh at least twenty-six stones," I said, not to be out-done. "You should try lifting her in and out of bed!"

But that didn't sound so dramatic. The surgical wards possessed the excitement and glamour of the popular television series, *Emergency Ward Ten*, and we imagined dealing with every drama and crisis that came our way.

Carol was on a male medical ward and had to shave men recovering from heart attacks.

"They're on warfarin to thin their blood," she said. "The problem is I keep nicking their skin with the razor. I can't get the bleeding stopped so I stick bits of tissue on their chins. What a sight they make for the doctors' round! I try to pretend it has nothing to do with me."

The ward round was an intimidating affair, conducted with great dignity. The consultants were eminent men who played the role of God to the junior staff. The medical team crowded into the ward, junior doctors and students bringing up the rear. They all wore white coats with stethoscopes sticking out of their pockets (nowadays they wear them casually draped round their necks.)

A complete hush prevailed during doctors' ward round. In the medical wards it often lasted an hour or more; patients and nurses alike were afraid to break the sacred silence. I took cover in the sluice and got on with the work there. If a patient needed a bedpan, or was sick, it made me feel marked for life as I tiptoed down the ward to attend to them. I was glad if another nurse got there first.

My main help in those early days came from a girl called Anna who was next on the ladder of seniority. She came from Keith in the North East of Scotland. She worked alongside me as we bed-bathed patients and gave them drinks. She showed me how to complete charts measuring patients' fluid intake, and how to record temperature and blood pressure readings. Once the sister thought I had gained a bit of competence she let me move on to more complicated procedures, such as giving injections, or dressing simple wounds.

Sometimes I was allowed to accompany the senior nurse on the medicine round. Medication was kept in a locked cupboard beside Sister's desk and she or the senior kept these keys pinned to their aprons, a mark of authority. The aura of this rubbed off on me as Nurse Clark and I set the trolley with bottles of mixtures, tablets, powders, medicine glasses and measuring spoons, not forgetting the bowl of warm soapy water to put glasses and spoons in after use before we washed them in the kitchen.

One lady whom Anna and I were very fond of on our medical ward was Mrs Docherty. She had been admitted in an extremely ill state with massive haemorrhaging caused by liver failure. She was a devout Catholic and received the last rites, but amazingly recovered and went home eventually. She had thick white hair and a thin, jaundiced face with enormous dark eyes. A lady on that first medical ward who was very different from Mrs Docherty was called Miss McGregor. She was ninety-two. In those days that was a remarkable age attained by few, but I remember her because she was such an old battle-axe! She was a retired hospital matron. She had trained in the same hospital some seventy years previously and never let us forget it. Her only visitor was the housekeeper she called her companion. This old woman in a maroon hat and coat seemed as ancient as Miss McGregor, but she was probably about twenty years younger.

Nothing ever pleased Miss McGregor. "You haven't dried my face properly, you used far too much soap. You haven't tucked that sheet in correctly."

"What a moan you are," I fumed to myself. Of course I couldn't say anything – after all who was the most important person in the hospital! But she really showed her true colours on Christmas Day.

I wondered what Christmas would be like. Women's magazines gushed over doctor and nurse romances and portrayed hospital Christmas full of festive cheer. If you believed them you would believe anything, we joked. What would the reality be like?

I decorated my room with festive sprigs of holly. On Christmas Eve, I had a split shift, so at two p.m. I went off duty for a couple of hours' break. Stuck to my mirror was a slip of pink paper. How nice, Home Sister had sent us all a message of goodwill! But no! With disbelief I read this curt order, "Nurse take these green twigs off the wall. If there are any marks on the newly painted wall you will be sent to Matron." Angry and near to tears I complied with the demand. I wished that some of my friends were around so that I could tell them about it, but it was later that night before we met together.

We were going to a midnight carol service in Glasgow Cathedral. We assembled in the Nurses' Home in our uniforms. Our navy cloaks with their red lining gave us a festive look appropriate to the season. We processed into Glasgow's ancient High Kirk. All my anger and hurt melted in the beauty of those mediaeval arches, soaring to the vaulted ceiling, their glorious stonework enhanced by the light of hundreds of candles. The service was televised and shown on black and white screens throughout Scotland. We nurses sat together, so the cameras often focused on us. I was amazed that many months later patients and their visitors said to me, "I ken who you are, hen, I saw you on the telly amang a' thae nurses."

That Christmas morning a crowd of us got up at six and went carol singing round the wards, still dimly lit before the rush of the new day. I'd never seen my ward in the subdued night lighting – it added to the atmosphere of stillness and peace. When we came on duty after breakfast, the ladies told us how much they'd appreciated the singing. Some of them were in tears.

"Och, hen that was grand," said Mrs Docherty. "There was me lying in bed missing my weans and in you came."

"It was just like the heavenly angels," added Miss Smith with a smile.

There was only one dissatisfied customer.

"And guess who that was," I told Anna when she came on for the late shift.

"Dinna tell me, It was that auld wifie, McGregor," Anna lapsed into her north east speech. "There's nae pleasing some folk at a'."

So we had a laugh at the sour old woman.

"She said it was a disgraceful performance. 'Who organised that?' she said to me when I was putting her on a bedpan. *She* said we should have marched smartly into the ward two by two instead of straggling in. Does she think we're in the army? Anyway," I went on, "we got so busy I didn't have time to worry about her. That lady who was admitted last night died at ten a.m. The two seniors did the body, so I was left to do all the temps and blood pressures and see to all the teas. I've been hectic. I hope it's quieter for you. Happy Christmas!"

So my first experience of hospital Christmas showed that life and death went on as usual whatever the season.

It wasn't customary to visit patients after their discharge, but one day while we were making beds Anna said to me, " Margaret, you remember Mrs Docherty? It would be fine to visit her. What would you think if we both tried to find her house? Have you any idea where she stays?"

"That's a great idea, Anna. I know where she lives. She's from Moodiesburn Street in Blackhill. I noticed her address because I live across the road."

The next week I'd finished work at 5p.m. and Anna had been off at 3.30, so we put our plan into action. It was dark in the early days of January. Yellow neon lights cast an eerie glow over the grey, three storeyed tenements of Blackhill. Groups of little girls bounced balls against the wall, or skipped in and out of an old clothes rope. Boys clattered metal hoops along the pavements to the accompaniment of barking dogs and the cry of 'Co-al, co-al briquettes!' The man selling the briquettes flicked the reins across the back of his old horse. His cart rattled along, carrying bricks of coal dust to people too poor to buy proper coal for the fires, their only means of heating.

A gang of teddy boys with drainpipe trousers, jackets with padded shoulders and winkle-picker shoes wolf-whistled as Anna and I crossed the road from the trolley bus stop. We quickened our pace. The wind blew greasy chip papers around our feet as we hunted for the open close and climbed dimly lit stone stairs to the third floor. Mr Docherty opened the door.

"Sure, lassies, it's great to see you. Come away in. Herself will be delighted to see you." Mrs Docherty was still thin and pale, but the jaundiced colour had gone.

"Och, nurses, I'm so pleased you've come to visit me," she said.

We all laughed at the term 'Nurses'.

"We're not being nurses now, just friends," said Anna.

So we all enjoyed a good evening together, drinking cups of tea and being served cheese slices on plain white bread by Kathleen, the fourteen-year-old daughter. The younger boys and girls crowded round wondering who we were. We looked so different out of uniform and away from the hospital ward. The fire warmed our faces and we chatted away until the clock on the mantelpiece chimed nine.

We caught the trolley bus back to the hospital along Royston Road, past old black tenements with shop windows boarded up.

"They have to barricade the windows like that to stop burglars," I told Anna. "My granny's newsagent's was up the hill from here. It was broken into regularly because two goods trains went by together at one o'clock in the morning and that's when they got in to steal cigarettes."

"I'm glad that it's nae like that in Keith," Anna replied. "No one ever locks their front doors. You know, it was great to see Mrs

Docherty in her own home. Folk are just bodies in the bed in the hospital.'

I agreed with her. Perhaps that was when the idea of working as a district nurse first took root in my mind, although it would be more than twenty years before I would actually begin that phase in my life. At eighteen I couldn't look so far ahead. For now, I was moving on to night duty on a male surgical ward. New challenges lay ahead.

Chapter 3: Cut throat Razor and Coddled Eggs

"Pack bags everybody, we're on the move," Carol announced. "The change list is up and we're on night duty as from Sunday. We've to sleep out at the Home in the infectious diseases hospital, you know the one beside the Celtic football ground. All right for you, Joan, you're a great Celtic fan."

"Aye we'll maybe get to see the game," Joan laughed.

"Don't be daft – we'll be asleep on Saturday afternoons," we told her.

"That's a pity. Why are we going away out there?"

"Home Sister says it's quieter and we'll sleep better," Carol said. "We go there on the hospital bus. By the way I like your hair, Joan, you really suit that style."

"Thanks. I was needing a new perm. It's much easier to keep tidy. Sister Mack was always girning on about my hair. I'm going to Ward Nine and I want to impress my new patients," Joan patted her fashionable bouffant style.

"Not just the patients," Carol teased. "Doctor Gordon, the resident on that floor is drop-dead gorgeous."

"Fantastic! I'll knock him up at two a.m. when somebody's drip runs through."

"Don't kid yourself, your senior will do that. You won't get a look in."

"Och, you never know, she might be away to her dinner," replied Joan as we went away to pack.

On my first spell of night duty, I was on a male general surgical ward. It was the first time I'd nursed men. No nice scented soap and talcum powder, just imperial leather soap and the occasional Old Spice after-shave. There were far fewer flowers in a male ward, a good thing from the junior nurses' point of view because flowers were taken out of the ward each night, lined up in their vases in the corridor, and brought in again in the morning. Although thick Glasgow smog polluted the winter air, it was thought that carbon dioxide given off by the flowers at night might be bad for our patients, so out the dahlias, daffodils, carnations and chrysanthemums had to go.

A female ward had so many flowers it took ages to trail them in and out, and there were complaints from the ladies if they didn't get their own flowers back beside their beds in the morning. The men didn't worry about such niceties.

The first night on duty, I came into the ward at nine o'clock on Sunday evening. Sister Jones gave Mary, the senior nurse and me the report, went off the ward and left us to start settling the patients for the night.

"This is the first time I've been in a male ward," I confided to Mary, who turned to me with a smile.

"Don't worry, we'll work away together and you'll be fine,"

We went round the patients, tucking them in for the night. Old Mr Hickey at the top of the ward had been admitted with a hernia, but was found to be suffering from scurvy, a result of impoverishment and malnutrition. This was early 1961. Lonnie Donnegan was hitting the big time with skiffle, and red haired Lulu went from Dennistoun to the Top of the Pops. Where were the swinging sixties for this old man? Before he could go to theatre he had to have his general condition improved. Scurvy would cause bleeding so he was a poor subject for surgery.

He used to sit up in bed in the middle of the night peeling oranges for his vitamin C supplement, the recognised treatment for scurvy since the days of Admiral Nelson. As he sucked at his oranges with his toothless gums he made good use of the wee small hours by sharpening his cut-throat razor on a leather strap. At first I wondered what the rustling and swishing noises were at two o'clock in the morning. The ward was lit with a green shaded night-light, and we had a similar light on the desk where we wrote reports and filled in charts. Looking up, it took a minute for your eyes to adjust to the darkness. I would tiptoe up to Mr Hickey's bed. "Shsh," I would whisper loudly because his hearing wasn't too good. "You'll wake up the other men."

"Sure, darlin' I'm after getting my vitamins," he'd whisper back even more loudly. "An' I'm just making sure my razor's sharp enough so I don't cut myself in the morning. Feel the blade I've put on it now."

One night just before we put the lights out for the night we became aware of a smell of burning.

"Nurse, where's the nurse? Nurse, call the fire brigade! We're gaunnae burn in our beds," yelled three or four voices together as Mary and I rushed across the ward. We knew who the culprit was because old Pop Ferguson always smoked his pipe in bed and we were forever scooping charred matchsticks from between the sheets.

"I'm awfy sorry, lassies, I must hae nodded aff," he confessed. "But the bed's no' gone up in flames, it's only a wee bit scorched."

"Aye, but what's Sister Jones going to say when she sees that big brown singed hole in your counterpane," scolded Mary with a twinkle in her eye. "She'll give you a good skelping."

"Don't worry, Mr Ferguson, we'll stick this counterpane in the laundry basket and once it's been to the wash Sister will never know whose bed it came from," I said. I told Mary about Sally's burnt pillow at the pre-nursing school. "I'm getting good at hiding the evidence."

The ward specialised in the strange-sounding peripheral vascular disease – narrowing of the blood vessels. One man, a retired general practitioner, had his leg amputated. He suffered phantom pains and became so addicted to methadone he kept shouting, "Where's the Nurse? Bring my methadone at once." With him and Mr Hickey, the night watches were far from peaceful.

At first when Mary went for her meal break at three a.m. and I was left alone in the ward, I thought something dire would happen. When she came back I said, "All the men are still lying peacefully in bed, it's just as well they don't know that their lives have been in my hands! I should have asked Doctor Taylor to come and keep me company."

"Good idea," Mary replied. "Though I don't think he would be too happy – he's worked seventy-two hours non-stop already and there will be loads of new admissions tonight."

Sometimes it seemed as though the whole of Glasgow's stabbings and slashings were admitted to our ward on Saturday night, especially when there was a Rangers and Celtic game and bottles and knives flew freely.

Mary escorted a team of doctors round the new admissions, while I looked after patients still coming up from Casualty. We had already prepared receiving beds. Four months before I had been learning this in college with Joan or Sally tucked into the bed. Now I was on my own and it was for real. Men were brought in with perforated duodenal ulcers, writhing in acute pain and vomiting blood. Children were admitted with appendicitis, frightened and crying with pain and shock. These were the usual sights on receiving night but we also had to deal with patients mutilated after horrific mining and road accidents.

Two porters lifted each badly injured man on a stretcher from the hospital trolley. "One, Two, Three, Lift" and there was the casualty lying on the bed before he had time to blink. They slid the long stretcher poles out of the canvas, and I rolled the patient over as they pulled the canvas out from underneath him. In hospital every one is part of the drama of life and death and the porters always boosted the patients' morale with a laugh and a kind word.

"You'll be fine noo Jimmy, this young lassie will see you aw right," they would say.

Then off they'd go with the empty trolley ready for the next admission.

As the beds filled up porters wheeled extra beds from the store and lined them down the middle of the ward. Mary and I carried screens up and down to try to give a modicum of privacy. At five a.m., still in the half-light we started the daily routine of nursing care for the very sick, washing and changing severely injured patients before switching the main ward lights on at six o'clock. We checked temperatures, pulses, blood pressures and respirations. Mary went round with the medicine trolley and I trundled the bathing trolley to men who were bed-bound. Our shift ended with the ward report when the day staff came on duty at eight o'clock.

I met up with my usual crowd at breakfast. The day nurses had left for their shift and we swapped stories over scrambled eggs on toast in the half empty dining room.

"You should have seen my ward last night,' I said. 'It was like a battlefield. A guy was brought in with his legs sliced to bits.'

"No – what had happened?" the others asked.

"He works down the pits. He got caught in the coal-cutting machine. I tell you, it was really gruesome. There was blood everywhere. He was in theatre all night. And there was this other boy, he's only twenty. He came off his motor bike. He's in a complete coma. I had to put ice packs on his head – his eyes were so swollen.'

"That's awful. There's no hope for him, I suppose. I had someone in a coma too," said Joan, fresh from her first medical ward. "She's only eighteen like us and she's diabetic. Remember Miss Black going on about how their urine smells like fresh mown hay – well, it does! I just couldn't believe it."

"Colour of normal urine, pale amber and clear…" Sally recited, quoting our college notes. "And for examination the nurse must note colour, smell, reaction and specific gravity. But, look, we're having our breakfast, let's talk about something else."

"Breakfast, don't remind me," Carol groaned.

"Why, what's the matter?" we asked.

"Well you know how we have to cook the eggs for the patients' breakfast on Sunday mornings? These young guys in my ward got me into a right tiz. One asked for his egg to be boiled for one minute, another said, 'Two minutes, please, nurse.' And the third one asked for his to be done for three minutes, and even then I didn't realise something was up. I was so worried I'd get it wrong I made Mum test out all the different times at home and then I phoned her from the call box in the Nurses Home to find out how she was getting on."

We all laughed.

"They were pulling your leg," said Joan, "But you'll never guess what I was asked. This woman in my ward demanded a coddled egg!"

We looked mystified. We'd heard about coddling people but not eggs.

"Even Miss Black didn't tell us about that," Sally said. "Although she made out she knew everything."

So we spent our nights on duty and our days sleeping out in the Home to which we were bussed each morning. I felt tired and disorientated by the night shift, but as soon as I put my uniform on things fell back into focus and I felt able to face anything.

Three sisters went round the whole hospital every night. They expected us to know the names and conditions of the patients by heart. So we would mug it up. "Mr. Smith 1st postoperative day following an appendicectomy, Mr Stewart 2nd post-op day after a partial gastrectomy." Then there were all the amputations, were they below or above the knee, the right or left leg, and would Sister Mills remember better than I did? She would bustle into the ward during the night between one and four a.m. and expect you to drop everything, including the patient, and conduct her round. If the ward was going like a fun fair and the bed wheels were crooked or the curtains not neatly pulled back, she would let you know about it. People could be rushed to theatre for emergency surgery, relatives could be anxiously waiting outside the door, blood and guts and gore had flowed freely all night; none of that seemed to matter. Sister Mills' priority was order and discipline.

No matter how hectic the night had been senior student nurses had to present a full written report for the day sister.

"Mr. Black was in theatre for a choledochojejunostomy. He's got a drain in situ to be removed in four days. No soakage from the wound."

Now how could you write that at seven a.m. with so much else to do? So you wrote it earlier and had to alter things: 'Mr Stuart had a good night and slept well – but died at 5a.m.'

Deaths occur more frequently at night. One morning Joan told us there had been so many deaths that she heard the porter singing "Gin a body meet a body," as he trundled his trolley into the ward yet again.

Romance was in the air for Joan and her "drop-dead gorgeous" resident doctor.

We kept hearing stories about Kenny Gordon. One night ever-so-fabulous Kenny and Tommy the porter hoisted Joan into the trolley used for bodies. She laughed about it when she told us the tale but it hadn't seemed so funny at the time.

"I nearly wet myself, I was so scared," she confided. "I thought they were going to wheel me down to the morgue! But I got my own back."

"What could you do to cap that?" Sally asked.

"My senior, Jeanette said Kenny's fond of chocolates, so we got some mersalyl, you know the stuff the patients get as a diuretic? We injected an ampoule into his favourite Dairy Box."

"The poor guy would have to run to the loo day and night," we laughed.

With escapades like this the three months' night duty passed quickly. Now it was back to the classroom for a month. Each weekend would be free and we could catch up on normal sleep.

Chapter 4: Love and Loss

Back in the classroom for junior nursing lectures and exam we met up with the rest of the crowd from the probationary course. By now nearly everybody had started to smoke. Sally struggled hard to master the technique.

"Sally, why on earth do you bother, you're obviously not enjoying it," I said.

"It's all right for you, Margaret, you've never started. Go on, have one," said Sally, offering her packet of Senior Service.

"No thanks, I took a puff once. It made me feel so horrible I've never wanted to try again."

One of our practical subjects was bandaging. Soon we were adept at spiralling crepe in figures of eight up and down our arms and legs, fingers and thumbs: if it went up it was called ascending spica, descending spica if it went down. We bandaged each other's heads, eyes, ears, hands and feet. We learned to do a mastectomy bandage and a stump bandage.

We were taught to make poultices – linseed, starch and kaolin. The only one actually in use in the wards was kaolin. It was used to reduce inflammation if the contents of an intravenous infusion had leaked into the tissues surrounding the veins. We were taught the theoretical use of leeches, making us feel decidedly mediaeval. These small worms manufacture a powerful anti-coagulant to encourage bleeding and also suck out infected material from the wound.

The dressings materials used in wound care had strange sounding names like gutta percha tissue, jaconet and oiled silk.

"It sounds like we're going fishing," Carol remarked. "You catch a perch with your net and wear oilskins to keep out the wet," she chanted.

"Hey, dig the poetry!" Joan put in.

Nursing in those days was an art based on established tradition. We learnt facts and practical skills without asking questions. The patients were not encouraged to ask questions either. Is that why they were called patient?

Once the exam was over we went back on day duty, but now, nine months into our training our original crowd was smaller. One girl left to be married. The shift pattern and compulsory residence in the Nurses' Home made it impossible for a married woman to carry on with nursing training. Some girls had developed back problems and were compelled to give up and one or two had decided that nursing was definitely not for them.

The rest of us went on through our training. Joan's romance was going strong with Dr Kenny. Carol was dating one of his friends, I had fallen in love with David, an engineering student, and Sally had met a handsome young policeman during her time in Casualty.

"Roddy's very musical," she said. "He plays in the Police Band."

"Kenny is too," said Joan. "He really likes the cello. We went to a symphony concert last week. What does your man play?"

"Well, actually," Sally confessed. "It's the big drum. He's six foot two, they picked him for the drum because he can see over the top."

We fell about laughing and Sally chuckled too. "Never mind," she said. "You keep in with me because Roddy's from Lewis and he can get us tickets for the dance at the Highlanders' Institute. Who's off to the jigging?"

We laughed again, but then I remembered pretty little Anne Marie.

"Oh, girls, I said, "we can go dancing, but this wee girl was admitted the other day. She'd been run over by a car."

"Oh no," my friends exclaimed. "Was she badly hurt?"

"She's had her leg amputated. She'd loved Highland dancing and that's what reminded me. She's only nine and now her dreams are over. The resident was almost in tears when he had to break the news to her Mum and Dad."

Little Anne Marie was the only child in the adult ward and the ladies who were up and about enjoyed making a fuss of her.

"There, doll, you're a wee star," they would tell the pretty wee girl when they'd piled her black curls high on her head.

"She's getting on so well," I said to Anna whom I met in the dining room one day. We hadn't seen each other for months, and it turned out Anna was about to go on to my ward for her final spell on night duty. "You'll love her. She's very brave. She's already running around on her artificial leg."

"Aye, children can be so brave," Anna said. "There was this wee lassie I nursed in the Burns Unit. She was only four, and you wouldna believe what happened to her. Some boys wrapped newspapers round her and set her alight. She was covered in burns from head to foot!"

"That's really awful. How could anyone do such a thing? Is she getting any better?"

"I got moved away from that unit so I never found out the end of the story. Mind the time we went to see Mrs Docherty?"

"Yes, but we never managed to go back," I said. "I went on night duty, you went away for your fevers' block and we haven't really seen each other since."

"That's how it goes," Anna said, philosophically. "By the way, I've applied to Raigmore for my midwifery."

"Raigmore? Oh, up in Inverness. That's near to Lossiemouth. I've met this gorgeous guy who belongs there."

"So you're going out wi' a Lossie loon! That's fine! I'll maybe see you if he takes you up to meet his folks." We both agreed on that, but once Anna had moved away we never saw each other again.

In the same ward as Anne Marie was a lady with terminal cancer. Mrs Wishart was so uncomplaining although her condition was rapidly deteriorating. There was so little we could do for her but she still appreciated small things like her own pretty nighties and fragrant talcum powder and soap.

"My hands always smell so nice after I've helped you wash," I'd say and she'd smile with pleasure.

One day, a neighbour from her Bridgeton tenement, sharing the same stairhead toilet was admitted to the bed opposite. She was an emergency patient with a festering carbuncle and Mrs Wishart was very distressed to see her.

"Oh no, no' that yin," she whispered. "She's bad for the drink and you dinnae want to hear her language. I never thought I'd end my days with her opposite my bed," she added in tears.

I didn't know what to say. I realised that she had guessed the truth we'd all kept hidden from her. However, within a day or two Mrs Wishart was moved: her bed was wheeled into the side ward to enable her to die in privacy.

Dying patients were cared for in this way. Doctors on the ward round walked past their beds, unable to offer any hope. It was out of this that the hospice movement developed when Dame Cicely Saunders realised that the physical, emotional and spiritual needs of dying patients and their families were not being met in general hospitals.

This was especially the case when a child died. I nursed Andrew, a little boy of three, suffering from leukaemia. Today there is an 80% success rate in the treatment of childhood leukaemia, but in the early 1960s there was very little anyone could do and we knew that this dear little boy had only six weeks at most to live. One morning I dressed him up in my cap and apron and carried him round the ward.

"Here's our new nurse," I announced.

The men round about gave him a wave and a smile. Andrew was the only child in the ward. I went off duty for three nights, and when I came back I saw an empty bed where Andrew had been. The book in which deaths were recorded was lying open on the desk and there was wee Andrew's name. I felt very distressed but no more was said. I've often thought about this since. We were trained not to show our feelings and yet how can we suppress emotion and still be good nurses?

Working in my local hospital meant that sometimes people whom I knew were admitted as patients. Towards the end of my second year a teacher from my secondary school was admitted with kidney failure.

I wanted to visit him, but Sally, who was nursing him, dissuaded me. "Mr Craig is very confused and agitated," she said.

"Oh that's terrible, I don't want to see him then," I said. "He was such a great teacher. I'd rather remember him how he was."

"He needs dialysis," Sally said. "But you know what it's like, there's only a limited number of kidney machines."

"Yes, and Mr Craig's a bachelor – we could never understand it. Half the girls in the class had a crush on him."

Sally and I both knew that a middle-aged bachelor would not rate as a priority for dialysis. In a hospital life and death are so much part of the daily routine that our talk soon moved on to other topics.

"I'm being moved to male orthopaedics next week," I told Sally. "Remember when Carol was there, and they kidded her on, making her boil all those eggs? These guys on traction for weeks have nothing else to do but wind us up."

"Yes, you watch out," Sally cautioned. "Pyjama trousers don't go over the weights and pulleys so they wear bikini bottoms. They'll ask you to tie the tapes on. 'I cannae dae it mysel, hen. Gonnae gie's us a haun,' they'll say."

"Thanks for warning me. At least we'll get a laugh, not like those old grannies with their fractured femurs in the female ward."

Old ladies who had fractured the neck of their femurs were frail and often confused. Many had raised big families in cramped tenement flats and were very unwilling to get up and walk with crutches. "Oh hen, jist leave me in ma bed the day," they groaned.

"How's orthopaedics, Margaret?" Carol asked later.

"Oh, I'm getting on fine there, and the young lads Sally was going on about are great. But there's one man who thinks he's so smart. You know how you have to ask them every day when you do the temps, 'have your bowels moved today'? Well, he says, 'They've moved to Ardrossan, they've moved to Carnoustie, they've moved to Edinburgh.' Does he really think he's being a laugh? Once maybe, but not every day. He's beginning to get me down."

"He sounds a real pain. You should give him a soap and water enema, high hot and helluva lot. That would move him somewhere all right, double quick!"

So, as in any hospital, all human life was there. There was also animal life – patients were admitted with lice. In fact all emergency patients were admitted into blankets on top of the bed. They had to be scrubbed thoroughly and their toe and fingernails cleaned and cut before being lifted into clean sheets. The shock of this was too much for some and they expired rather ungratefully.

"At least they went out clean," we consoled ourselves. And we could show off our handiwork to the ward sister, pleased that she couldn't find fault with the spotless body lying on the bed.

Which brings us to those stalwarts of the Old Hospital regime, Florence Nightingale re-incarnated, the dreaded ward sisters.

Chapter 5: Strict Sisters and Glamour Girls

The time has come to talk about the sisters who ruled their domain with a rod of iron. They were unmarried ladies who had worked in the same ward for so long they seemed in with the bricks, as cold and hard as the long white tiled corridors they stalked along to reach their fiefdom.

Everything and everyone was put firmly into place. The junior doctors certainly came in for criticism. I heard one sister grumble, "Young man, you've left the desk in a mess with all these blood tubes lying around. Put them away as soon as you've finished with them, please."

The fact the said young man had been out of his bed for the last thirty-six hours made no difference. The ward had to be run like a ship, with Sister the captain and every student nurse had to be licked into shape under her stern command. She would criticise our untidy hair and general appearance, despite the fact we'd been running up and down the ward for eight hectic hours. "Nurse, look at the state of your shoes, they're worn through. How dare you come on to my ward looking like that? Go and purchase a new pair on your day off this week."

The litany of complaints continued.

"Why is the linen cupboard so untidy, the bed wheels not all facing in a line down the ward or the screens not straight, and as for the bed pan trolley, well it's a disgrace! Where's that nurse? Why are you talking to the patient in bed 3? Go and tidy the sluice."

Some of these women were eccentric in the extreme. Sister Dunn never took her day off when the off-duty sheet said she should, so neither the nurses nor patients could relax. The atmosphere in her ward was tense and unhappy with patients, nurses and even the visitors worrying they would step out of line. One man made the terrible mistake of dying when his bed was at the top end of the ward, rather than being neatly hidden away at the bottom. Sister covered his face with a sick bowl and made the nurses wheel the bed down the ward, whilst she spoke to the corpse, "Never mind, Mr. Smith, you'll be better soon. Once we've moved you down the ward a bit you'll come on like a house on fire." The other patients pretended not to notice the dead man's hand drooping over the covers, and his totally still body.

I was sent to Sister Dunn's ward for my first senior medical night duty.

"Oh, gosh, I'm so glad I'm going there on nights, at least I'll only see her for a short time before she goes off duty, and again in the morning," I said when we were looking at the change list.

"That's what you think, Margaret. Sister creeps back into the ward at all hours of the day or night," Joan replied. "You can never be off your guard for a minute."

"That horror, I never want to see her again," Sally said in tones of utter conviction. " She terrorised me when I was there that first trial week in the wards. It was only you lot who stopped me leaving then."

In Sister Dunn's ward patients with heart attacks were kept on a very strict diet as Sister reckoned they would improve more quickly. Two men in neighbouring beds, both recovering from a coronary thrombosis started a conspiracy with the night nurses.

"Now, Nurse, we've got a couple of eggs each here. You take them into the kitchen for us, and then at two o'clock in the morning we'd like you to make us scrambled eggs on toast. We always have a cup of tea then and the last nurses obliged us with this treat. We're starving to death here, you know," Mr Brown put on such a doleful face I had to laugh.

"Whatever would Sister say? My life won't be worth living if she found out," I protested.

"Don't worry, we keep our eyes open for her coming. She's never caught us yet."

So Mr Brown and Mr Moffat sat up in bed every night enjoying their scrambled eggs. Whether they got better more quickly as a result I don't know, but their little rebellion brightened up their lives and gave them a break from the boredom of the strict regime that Sister insisted upon.

Sister Gibb doted on her goldfish and the potted plants she kept on the broad wooden window sill in her room. It was rumoured that she gave the fish oxygen to prolong their lives. When she was on holiday and the fish or plants died the nurses rushed around the shops trying to find a good match.

"Was that goldfish all one colour or did it have some white markings on it?" wondered Carol, when she and one of the other nurses on the ward were given the onerous task of replacing yet another of Sister Gibb's fish.

"I wanted to write in the night report. 'Goldfish's condition deteriorated during the night because the nurses were too busy with real patients,' " Carol continued. "Of course I didn't dare. But wait till I tell you, the other night when we came on, all we could see was Sister's backside."

"Some view that would be, whatever was she doing?" I asked.

"She'd lost her gold tooth in the ward after her supper, and she was down on her hands and knees at the bottom of the ward looking for it in the cracks in the floor boards," Carol replied. "'You nurses will have to look for my tooth before you start the rest of the work', she told us."

"Did you find the tooth?" I asked.

"The lady in the first bed had an epileptic fit. We were too busy looking after her to worry about the daft old bat and her stupid tooth."

Sister Kerr was obsessed with how highly polished her desk was. It was the job of the junior night nurse to polish it each night until it gleamed. If Sister couldn't see her face in it when she came on duty in the morning, the nurse would be made to do it again before going off duty.

The most eccentric was Sister Hamilton. She insisted that all the bedpans were brought down from the sluice at 7.40 a.m. prompt and piled up on the piano, whose other use was to play the hymns when people from the local Gospel Hall held church services in the ward on Sunday evenings. The bedpans were put there for her to inspect to make sure they reached the level of cleanliness she deemed correct. The patients in her ward all knew that the needs of nature had to be held in check at that time in the morning.

I suppose most of these women had trained during the Second World War when nurses only got one day off a month. Innovative and proactive they were not, but these words were not part of the nursing vocabulary then. We felt they had no interest in the wellbeing of us students who were left to sink or swim.

"We're just numbers to these horrible women aren't we?" Sally said ruefully, and we had to agree.

Not all the sisters were like this, or none of us would have stayed the course. Sister Coutts was very correct in her royal blue uniform, her white starched apron immaculate and her hospital badge polished to perfection but Carol had a good story to tell.

"Sister Coutts is a character," she said. "The other day she was watching me shorten Mr Donald's drainage tube. Some bile leaked on to the floor. 'Oh no,' I thought, 'that's me failed my assessment.' But Sister said, 'See's a dod of cotton wool, hen'. She mopped up the spilt fluid and walked off up the ward."

"That's a bit like Sister Duncan in ward twelve," I said. "Yesterday evening there were just her and me on duty. I went and dropped six plates of shepherds' pie on the floor. You can imagine how I felt because that's all there was for the patients' suppers, but whilst I cleaned up the mess, she went into the kitchen and made scrambled eggs and toast for the ladies instead. I couldn't believe how nice she was."

"It's because you're still madly in love," teased Carol. "You were floating on air instead of holding on to the supper trolley."

I joined in the laughter. "Imagine if it had been that pernickety Sister Kerr and her polished desk. Mince on the floor would be the end for her."

You remember the good times and the bad, but I wonder how the patients we cared for remember us?

One nurse had a beautiful singing voice. In the evening she and I hurried through our work, then she sang to women who were all recovering from major surgery and worrying how their families at home were managing without them.

She sang the old favourites, Loch Lomond, Mhairi's Wedding, the Rowan Tree, By Cool Siloam's Shady Rill, The 23rd Psalm, The Old Rugged Cross. We listened spellbound. I'm sure those patients slept better and recovered quicker as a result.

Some of us must have been abrupt and uncaring at times. We had to deal with harrowing situations, and see grief and anguish suffered by patients and their families. I'm sure we weren't the angels nurses were euphemistically called.

My mother suffered from Parkinson's Disease and sometimes needed hospital treatment. She once asked, "Why do nurses always say 'Wait a minute'?" I tried not to say it after that, but the phone would be ringing, somebody was sick, a drip was running through, a thousand and one things were claiming my attention so I went back to the refrain, "Wait a minute."

During my training, I developed recurring bouts of tonsillitis, so the Home Sister sent me to the sick bay in the Nurses' Home.

"God, Margaret, this place is like a morgue," Carol exclaimed when she came to visit me.

"Home Sister runs this sick bay the way Miss Black taught us a ward should be run," I told her ruefully. "I tell you, Carol, I know how the patients feel now. The doctor's ordered intramuscular injections of penicillin four times a day. You feel the stuff going right down your leg. I can't tell you how sore it is!"

"Never mind Margaret, at least you're warm in here. Look at the smog outside. The wards are so busy with people with chest infections. There are so many wee babies with croup. We nurse them in those steam tents we learnt about in training school."

Glasgow was still a city afflicted by winter smog. Traffic came to a standstill. Until 1962 when the last old Glasgow tramcar made its final journey to Auchenshuggle, the tram lines were used by cars and pedestrians alike as a certain way of finding the way home. White nylon petticoats became a permanent grubby grey, black streaks ran down your face and neck from the wet sooty air, and when you blew your nose you realised what the contaminated atmosphere was doing to your lungs.

All the same we did our best to keep up with the style. You could find nurses having a good night out at the University Students' Union or the Highlanders' Institute. We went to the cinema occasionally and when funds were low we would sit in a café with our boyfriends, making a cup of espresso coffee last for the whole evening.

Where could you go to whisper sweet nothings in your lover's ear? I remember dark winter evenings going up the fire escape in the medical block. If Sister Dunn had looked out of her window and seen the Royal Infirmary equivalent of Juliet's balcony scene, I would neither have known or cared.

Then there was the annual ball, which was a grand affair in evening dress. Carol went with Andrew, the doctor she was dating, and Joan and Kenny made up a foursome. The next year Sally and I went with David and Roddy.

We wore long dresses, mine was black chiffon with a silver top. I'd been given a 3.30 finish that day, so I rushed to the hairdresser's and had my hair brushed in the bouffant style so fashionable in the sixties. We hired a taxi from the hospital and saw Joan looking out from her ward window to wave us off as we left in style.

Our annual leave was mostly at lovely times like November and February. Where were you when President Kennedy was assassinated? I was on holiday visiting relations in England. On £9 a month I couldn't go very far.

Once we were lucky to have a week's holiday in the summer time. Sally and Joan went off to Arbroath. Sally won the Miss Arbroath bathing beauty contest.

"Such a claim to fame!" we declared when they showed off the pictures in the local newspaper.

"My nose was all sunburnt, I never thought I had a chance," Sally told us.

"But you're nice and tall, that's what models are supposed to be like. Miss World had better watch out!" said Carol

When Sally was being feted in the local paper, I went hiking in the Lake District with a cousin who was a nurse in London. She introduced me to the culinary delights of Vesta packets of dried Chinese chop suey, chow mein and fried rice, which we cooked for our evening meal in the Youth Hostel.

We enjoyed comparing experiences of nursing life in London and Glasgow. Nurses in London sometimes got complimentary tickets for the theatre, which would have been rather fine.

Back in Glasgow, Carol and I once went out together for a meal. We got a surprise when we asked for the bill – it had already been paid. Someone who had been a patient in Carol's ward had seen us and without saying anything had paid our bill.

By now we all seemed to have a romance on the go and hearts were broken and mended. No nurse could be married until she had finished her training. Our lives were still restricted by the rules of the Nurses' Home, and by the late shifts we worked each week.

No wonder those dreaded sisters had never married! Hospital work for that earlier generation had made off duty life almost impossible. But now we must go back to the wards…

Chapter 6: Finishing the Course

As a senior student nurse I worked in the cardiac unit where I had the opportunity to see surgery performed by a famous surgeon.

"It was incredible," I told Carol. " I watched the Professor open up the patient's mitral valve – you could actually see the heart beating."

"I enjoyed Cardiology too. It's great to be part of a team involved in pioneering work," she answered enthusiastically. "Open heart surgery means the difference between life and death, especially for kids with heart defects."

"They used to be called blue babies, like wee Stephen with a hole in his heart."

"He's a real wee fighter that one. So he's had his operation now?"

"Yes, I nursed him in intensive care," I said. "It's so different, all those machines and monitors. Sometimes you forget there's a person there, you're so busy looking after the equipment."

"Just the same, intensive care units are how things will go in the future," Carol replied.

After Cardiology I moved on to Casualty. In total contrast to the new technology in the cardiac unit, a First World War veteran hobbled up with shrapnel in his leg.

"I brought this hame frae the Somme," he explained. "I've read aboot thae new heart and lung machines in the *Sunday Post*, but, see this sair leg, they cannae mak it better. It's fair stoonin' the day."

"No wonder, it's so cold outside. They say this is the coldest January since records began." I said as I cleaned the pus from the wound sustained half a century ago.

"Ye're nae kidding. It's that's slippy, I couldnae keep my feet."

Next on the list was a victim of the severe cold. He was a fourteen-year-old boy with frostbitten fingers.

"Imagine seeing frostbite in Glasgow," I said to Carol over frothy coffee in the café down the road. "You'd think it was the North Pole! The skin was peeled right off his fingers as though he'd pulled off a pair of gloves."

"Gosh! I've never seen anyone with frostbite! However did he get like that?"

"He's a milk boy, they start the round at four in the morning. He doesn't wear gloves because he has to pick up the tokens, you know the ones people leave on the doorstep to pay for their milk? He can't get a hold of them with his gloves on, but then his fingers stuck to the glass bottles."

"You see everything in Casualty. I tell you, Margaret, it's like a battlefield on Saturday nights, razor fights, punch-ups and drunks with blood pouring from their heads. They vomit their guts up too!"

"Sounds just great," I replied. "But Sally met her hunky policeman there so it's got its attractions. How's your love life doing?"

"I'm going out with Bob. He's a smashing bloke. I met him at the Students' Union dance a couple of weeks ago."

"What's he doing, not a medic again?" I asked

"No, not this time. This one's studying architecture. He's in his fourth year. How's your romance going, Margaret?"

"I haven't seen much of David lately. It seems ages since I had a Saturday evening off."

"Well they say absence makes the heart grow fonder, how about another coffee?"

My third placement as a senior was orthopaedic theatre. I'd been looking forward to working in theatre, but orthopaedics seemed more like a carpenter's shop with the noise of hammers banging nails and plates into broken bones.

"I don't think I'm cut out for theatre," I told my friends. "I prefer the real nursing care on the wards. How about going into town tomorrow to cheer me up. I'm off from two to five, what about you?"

"I'll come with you," said Sally. "I've to buy my granny a birthday present. We get a good discount in Timothy White's don't we? I saw some nice talc for eleven and threepence and some cologne for eight and sixpence the last time I was looking round the shops."

"You'd better go now because next week we'll be back on nights," said Carol. "We won't be getting a suntan this summer, girls."

"The Arbroath News will have to look for a new pin-up girl this year, Sally," Joan laughed.

Our last months as students were spent working at night, sleeping during the day and trying to study for those important final examinations.

"What's the dose of epanutin, and what are the side effects?" we would ask each other at the meal break at three a.m., or "What are sulphonamides used for?"

"What on earth do you put on the trolley for a paracentis abdominis?" Sally would demand between gulps of tea. "There's so much to remember isn't there?"

"When you're busy at night with drips to set up, nasogastric tubes to pass, colonic lavages to do, and everything else as well, there's no time to worry about studying. I'm not going to bother," Joan said with bravado. "I need my sleep in the day."

It was Joan who gained the gold medal awarded to the best all round student of our year, so she must have been studying hard throughout our training, rather than leaving it to the last minute as some of us did.

The hospital final examinations lasted for two hours three days in a row. Each day we came off night duty at eight a.m., hurried home to snatch no more than three or four hours sleep in order to be in the exam room at three o'clock in the afternoon. Finally, in September, we were transferred back to day duty for a month before the final state examination, held as usual on our day off.

"Surely we could have an extra day!" we complained. Our senior tutor advised us to go to Matron with our petition. We looked at one another. Who would dare? The whole class voted. Joan and I were chosen for the grim task of confronting Matron with this unheard of request.

Matron glowered over the top of her spectacles. "Do you not realise that students have always sat their state examinations on their day off? No one has ever complained before. Where can we find more nurses to staff the wards? How can you possibly have the nerve to think that we should make a special case for you?"

There was no answer we could give. We made our escape, thankful to be on the other side of the door. Strangely enough, the following year the final students did get another day off. Perhaps our senior tutor had used us as pawns in a political game, but this was far from our thoughts as, still very shaken we hurried back to tell our friends.

The ward I worked in before my finals was the ear, nose and throat ward. It was very busy with children having their tonsils out. After they came back from theatre the wee souls were sick and miserable and had to be carefully monitored because of the risk of post-operative haemorrhage. There were also patients with mastoid infections, which could cause hearing loss. Patients with throat cancer had to have their larynx removed. They were wheeled to theatre, knowing they would never be able to speak again.

Two men were treated with a new drug called methotrexate. It was given in a drip intravenously, and had to run in at precisely eight drops a minute. I used to watch the drips like a hawk, concerned they would speed up and run in too fast. It was hoped that the drug would reduce the tumour, so that when surgery took place, it would be less extensive.

Some of the men with throat cancer couldn't swallow; their nutritional state was poor and they were very thin. We gave them switched egg and brandy which we poured down a nasogastric tube into their stomachs. We also gave bottles of stout the same way.

"This is the Cross Keys pub opening for business," I'd joke as I unlocked the medicine cupboard and took out the brandy.

"Cheers, hen, that's a fine drink ye're gieing me. Gaunnae poor oot anither yin," Mr Smith replied. It was the bright spot in his evening when he saw me coming towards his bed with a tray holding a glass of beaten egg or a bottle of Guinness.

There was a small emergency out-patient department attached to the ward. Children were often admitted to have beads or other foreign bodies, as the correct terminology went, removed from their ears or noses. They'd only stuck them up there out of curiosity – and now they were in hospital, with a nurse coming towards them with a big syringe with rubber tubing. I sat a wriggling three-year old on my knee, and used a solution of warm water and formaldehyde to syringe out the bead he'd poked in his ear. The solution had to be the correct temperature: too cold would cause dizziness and too hot would burn the child. The pressure of the syringe had to be maintained at a level that would not damage the eardrum. Eventually the ordeal was over and there was the red bead he'd been playing with floating in the bowl I held against his head.

"There, Tommy darling, you're all better now," I reassured him, before taking him tear-stained but happier, back to his anxious mother. She was not admitted into the treatment room during the messy procedure.

Whilst I was there the ward sister went off sick. I was left in sole charge of the ward. That would never happen now to an unqualified student.

In the midst of all this the final exams came almost as an anticlimax. We all passed and so now we were registered nurses and given our staff nurses' caps. Oblong in shape and stiffly starched, they had to be folded into pleats with a butterfly tail at the back. We were so proud of them. You had to walk with your head held high to keep them on!

"You look great in your staff nurse's cap, Margaret," Sally said admiringly in the changing room the first eventful day we put them on before going on duty.

"Thank you, so do you, Sally. We've come a long way since the preliminary training school. I wonder what Miss Black would say to us now."

"She'd say that your shoes need a good polish and your hospital badge is squint," Sally brought me down to earth again with a smile.

We wore our silver and blue hospital badge with pride. We'd worked hard for that badge. We'd cared for patients admitted in a diabetic coma, with coronary thrombosis, with strokes. We'd seen horrific wounds after road and work related accidents. Children had died of meningitis, leukaemia, pneumonia, and following surgery in our care. We'd also seen people admitted at death's door recover and go home. We'd nursed patients in the Burns and Plastics unit and seen skin grafting improve their disfigurements.

We all had memories of patients who had meant a great deal to us, showing courage and endurance, humour and patience in situations that we were still too young to appreciate properly. We had learnt to deal quickly and efficiently with anything that came our way. Nursing is hard work, as Granny had warned me before I started out, but the rewards of caring for people when they are vulnerable and distressed are immense. Now, with the confidence born of the last three years we looked forward to new responsibilities in our chosen career. Some of us stayed at the hospital for a year or so, working as staff nurses, but others including myself went on to do midwifery. A new chapter was beginning.

Chapter 7: Oil, Bath and Enema

"I'm applying to the Eastern District Hospital to do midwifery," I told my friends after the first excitement of qualifying was over.

"I thought I might go there too," Sally agreed.

"Well, I'm going to Rottenrow," Carol informed us. "After all, it's got the best reputation for midwifery."

"You have to wear a funny cap with a bow tied under your chin. I don't fancy myself in that at all," I objected. "I'm not into bows or anything frilly or fussy."

"You're too fussy yourself," Carol rejoined. "What about you Joan, where are you going?"

"I've applied to the Simpson's Maternity Hospital in Edinburgh. Kenny's got a senior registrar's job in the Western General there."

"So it's all change for a year at least," Carol concluded.

Rottenrow, the maternity hospital Carol had chosen is where obstetricians had pioneered Caesarean sections earlier in the century because so many women had developed misshapen pelvises as a result of childhood rickets. Public health had brought improvements, although the contraceptive pill was not yet prescribed extensively, and abortion was still illegal. When unmarried mothers were admitted in labour the sister gave them a wedding ring to wear during their stay in hospital. Without exception all the mothers were addressed as 'Mrs.' I soon discovered that some women came in for the seventh or eighth time. "I dinnae like tae see the cot empty beside my bed, hen, so I keep on falling wi' anither wean," one patient said, while a mother with seventeen children explained, "You see, dear, it's ma man's only pleasure, he disnae smoke or drink."

Women with all this experience of babies knew a lot more than I did my first day in a postnatal ward! I'd had no experience in handling newborn babies and was amazed at how tiny they were. I felt they would break in my hands, but there was no way you could let the mothers see how you worried you were. Sally and I both agreed that our general nurse training had given us the confidence to cope with this new situation.

There were only five students in the class. Sally and I, two other girls, red-haired Liz and Val with a soft Irish brogue. Unusually for that time there was an older lady, Anne, a missionary nurse in India, who had decided to take a year's leave and learn midwifery to enhance her skills.

Seeing my first baby being born was an emotional experience. I had tears in my eyes and Sally actually cried.

"I know I'm daft," she wept, "But it's all so beautiful."

Some of the mothers were frightened little girls who were younger than our twenty-one years. There were antenatal classes then, but it was not encouraged for the mother to take control of her labour, and no fathers were allowed to be present. The dreaded O.B.E. (Castor oil, a hot bath, and an enema) were prescribed to induce labour if the mother was overdue.

The postnatal wards were less enthralling than the delivery room because they had mums with the postnatal blues, mums with sore breasts, and babies with feeding problems. Mothers stayed in at least five days or longer, especially following a forceps delivery or a caesarean section.

There was an antenatal ward as well as the labour room and a special nursery for premature or sick babies. I especially enjoyed seeing the little premature babies develop. These little babies were red-skinned, with huge heads and eyes and their little bodies were covered in soft downy hair. Having been premature myself I felt quite an affinity for them, and now I understood why our mother always said that my twin sister and I had looked like skinned rabbits.

We had to tube feed babies who were slow to suck, and wash out the stomachs of babies who had swallowed mucus during the birth.

"Those wee mites needing to have their stomachs washed out are quite a handful aren't they?" Sally remarked.

"You need more than one pair of hands to pass the nasogastric tube, then pour water down the tube into its stomach, tip the tube into a bucket to let the stomach contents run out, and still keep a hold on the baby, " I agreed.

I always felt cruel doing it but it really helped to get these babies to feed properly. They stopped crying once it was all over and you gave them a cuddle.

It was very hot in the special nursery. We wore masks and gowns over our ordinary uniform. After a twelve-hour night shift you were exhausted with the heat as well as with the work. Sometimes the babies seemed exhausted too. They were so sleepy after the feed that I couldn't always get them to burp. Val coaxed the babies, "Come on you wee bugger, get that bloody wind up!" Her musical Irish voice worked wonders as they always obliged, lying happily up on her shoulder.

One baby in the nursery was an anecephalic, his head wasn't formed, and the brain and central nervous system had not been developed. This child lived for four days. The nursery nurse made him little caps out of gauze and kept him comfortable until he died.

"Oh, that's so sad," said Sally when I told her about him. "It's awful when something like that happens. The poor mother! I hope she has a healthy baby next time. Do you know what, Margaret, have you heard about the hypnosis classes in the ante-natal clinic?"

"Goodness, Sally, I thought that hypnosis only happened on the stage! Imagine it in a hospital!"

The consultant's self-hypnosis classes took place in the afternoon clinic. The ladies lay back in deck chairs, and the doctor taught them to relax so deeply that they were not aware of pain. We student midwives had to test the depth of their trance by injecting them with sterile needles. I was very interested in all this, but there was one drawback. We had to stand by the wall out of the way while the hypnotic voice repeated softly, "You're drifting away, you're drifting away."

"Margaret, you'll have to nudge me awake if I start to feel drowsy," Sally whispered one afternoon. "I ate too much steak and kidney pie at lunch for this."

I don't know how I didn't drift away too, even in my starched uniform. The women all enjoyed the experience. I saw two of them after they'd had their babies and asked how they'd got on. One had needed a forceps delivery and said she hadn't managed to hypnotise herself, although she'd drifted away perfectly peacefully in the clinic. The other mum had been more successful, and had got to the point when the baby's head was being born before she felt any pain.

There were ordinary relaxation classes in the clinic too, and classes to teach about labour and child care. Fathers didn't come. They were not expected to be present at the birth or have much to do with the infant once it was home. The women having their umpteenth baby didn't attend these classes. They knew it all backwards. But they were supposed to go to the clinic for the weight, urine and blood pressure tests, and also to have their abdomen palpated to find out the way the baby was lying, and to have the foetal heart rate measured. There were no ultra sound scans, but we got very practised in assessing the lie of the baby. The baby's heart was listened to using a thing like an ear trumpet. It was wonderful to hear it beating away. The first time I heard a heart beat this way I felt almost as emotional as seeing the baby being born, it was such an affirmation of new life.

The course was tough going with lectures after a twelve-hour night shift. Midwifery was often hectic, and if you were ever quiet in the labour ward, the sister in charge, an ex-army major insisted on you washing the walls of the labour room at three a.m. "Just to keep the troops occupied!" I thought as I wearily filled a bucket with hot water.

"Where's that student nurse gone to? There are walls to be washed before you skive off for your tea break," she'd shout.

At the end of six months I thought I would give it all up and go back to general nursing. I had a heart-to-heart talk with Sally in the dining room at three o'clock in the morning.

"Och, Sally." I said, "I don't think I'll do my second six months. I'd rather go back to general nursing."

Sally looked troubled, but then her hazel eyes flashed with determination.

"Don't be daft, Margaret," she remonstrated. "We've been through so much together, remember when I wanted to leave after that very first week on Sister Dunn's ward and how you all got me to change my mind? You kept me going then, so I'm not going to let you give up now. Besides," she went on, "The second six months will be better because the main exam will be over and the experience on district will be great."

She was right of course, and I was glad I followed her advice.

Help came from an unexpected source: my twin sister. I was feeling very tired and I badly wanted to use my nights off to visit my boy friend's family. David's father was in the merchant navy and was home for the first time in two years. I'd been invited to Lossiemouth to meet him, but the problem was I had lectures to attend. Instead of going away for a break I was supposed to trail back into the classroom. The good thing was you didn't have to wear uniform to attend the lectures, and my sister volunteered to go instead of me.

We planned our strategy in advance. My sister would meet Sally, Val and Anne, the missionary nurse, at the hospital gate.

"You'll have no problems recognising Jenny," I laughed.

"Let's hope nobody suspects," Anne sounded rather worried. "Should we be breaking rules like this?"

Anne was always very reserved. Looking back, I think she must have been in a culture shock, after her very different experiences in India, so now I tried to reassure her. "Don't worry, Anne. No one will notice because Jenny and I are very alike, even our boyfriends sometimes mix us up."

As it happened on the way through the gates, just as my sister had safely met with the other students, the first person to come along was the Matron, who asked, "Are you going to your lecture girls?" Fortunately she didn't realise there was an impostor in the midst!

"That was lucky," everyone sighed with relief. "Imagine meeting Matron – she's never usually around at this time of the morning!"

My sister scribbled pages of lecture notes. Afterwards I tried to make out her spelling of the unfamiliar medical terms.

"What's this word?" I wondered.

'Oh, I think the doctor said something like *physiogminy.* I didn't have a clue."

"I think he meant episiotomy," I said.

"Whatever's that?" she asked.

"Well perhaps you'd rather not know, but it's when they cut the vaginal opening to let the baby come out without the mother tearing," I informed her.

"Ouch, that sounds painful! Do you know, I couldn't believe you all stood up when that doctor came in, and you called him 'Sir'."

"Well that's how it is in nursing," I said. "Look, what's all this with *breach* written there?"

"He was going on about the baby lying the wrong way up. He kept pulling a doll through a pelvis and I pictured the baby breaching the birth waters into life. "

"You're hopeless! It's called *breech*, as in breeches because the baby's bottom comes out first. Your trouble is you read too much Shakespeare. 'Once more unto the breach, dear friends' isn't part of our coursework."

"I'd rather read Shakespeare than all that stuff, but it was interesting learning things you've spoken about so much."

So the time passed, I delivered baby after baby and each time felt the wonder of birth, sometimes tinged with sadness if the baby was unwanted or showed signs of being handicapped.

I still remember a red headed girl of eighteen who gave birth to a Down's Syndrome baby. He was her first baby and she was so shocked and upset. She lived in an old one- roomed tenement flat, and seemed so young and vulnerable. I've wondered over the years how she and her baby fared.

Most mothers though were excited as well as exhausted by their experience, even after several confinements. I can still hear the midwives' encouraging, "Here's a strong contraction, push down hard, keep it coming, keep it coming, push, push, *push*! Now stop pushing, pant, pant, the head's coming," then the cries of delight from the mother and the yelling of the baby making an undignified entry into the world. The labour ward was full of drama!

Our midwifery training required us to deliver ten babies in hospital and ten in their own homes in the community.

"I'm looking forward to going on district," I told my friends after a lecture about district midwifery.

"I think it will be lovely to deliver babies in their own homes," Sally agreed. "Birth's a natural occurrence after all."

"I was born at home," Val said. "It was war time when we were born, but our mums still managed, didn't they?"

Plenty of women gave birth at home in a situation very different from the sterile environment of the labour ward. Toilets on the stair and a sink with a cold water tap, only one or two rooms for the whole family, these housing conditions were common in Glasgow in the first part of the 1960s.

The Corporation provided the mothers with an allotted number of sheets of brown paper for the protection of the bed during the confinement. The brown paper sheets were burnt afterwards on the coal fire. You had to burn the placenta too after you'd examined it, in case the pet cat or dog got there first and ate it.

The midwife in charge of the delivery always needed at least four copper pennies in case she had to find a public phone to summon the flying squad, who came out to deal with an emergency. She also kept some shillings handy for the gas meter so that the gas and air machine wouldn't run out when it was most needed for pain relief.

The main office for the district midwives was in an imposing building owned by Glasgow Corporation in Ingram Street. This was in the city centre, an area connected with the tobacco lords of the eighteenth century when the city of Glasgow was growing from a village centred round St Mungo's Cathedral, to a thriving town. The midwifery office was in one of the mansions built by the nouveau riche of yesteryear.

We were given the names and addresses of the people we were to visit and set off from there. I was sent to the south side of Glasgow, a new area for me. I travelled through Kinning Park and the Gorbals wearing the midwifery student uniform of navy raincoat and a round hat. In today's hatless era this seems overdressed, but when you travelled without a car, braving wind and rainy weather, a hat was a real necessity, not just a fashion accessory. Whether the uniform was smart or antiquated, at that time in Glasgow a nurse could go anywhere and be perfectly safe.

"You'll never guess what happened," Sally told me excitedly one morning when we were in the office to be given our day's work. "I went to do a delivery in Roystonhill. I was just going into the close, hanging on to my hat to stop it being blown away, you know how the wind whistles round those closes, when all of a sudden, there were a couple of gangland heavies coming up to me. One of them had a huge scar down the side of his face. I thought my last hour had come."

"No wonder!" I breathed. But all had been well. The gang had greeted Sally with genuine smiles. "Ye'll no' meet wi' ony hairm, hen," they had reassured her. "The wumman ye're gaun tae steys on the second flair. We'll tak you back doon the stair again efter."

To reach my district I travelled on the Glasgow underground train system, called the subway. I glided down the Buchanan Street Station escalators deep underground, breathing in that distinctive smell of recycled air and travelled under the Clyde to Kinning Park Station. I walked along Scotland Street, past the local school designed by Charles Rennie Mackintosh, feeling perfectly at ease, despite the deprivation all around. Nurses were held in high esteem by the ordinary folk of Glasgow. I walked through places that were designated as slums, meeting nothing but kindness and helpfulness if I needed to ask directions to a street or tenement.

Once I went to a tenement in Florence Street in the Gorbals to attend a delivery. When we were going to a confinement, the Corporation of Glasgow provided a car to take us to the house, so that we could be sure of reaching the mother in time. That day there were no ordinary cars available so I was driven to the house in the Lord Provost's car, seated in grandeur in the back seat. I arrived at an eighteenth century smoke-blackened tenement. It was pulled down soon after in the upheaval of the Gorbals modernisation programme. On the pavement, watching the car draw up, a crowd of little children had gathered ready to wave to the Queen whom they thought must have been visiting in this official limousine.

"That's no' the queen," one of them said in disappointment.

"It's a nurse wi a black bag. Maybe it's got a baby inside. Ma maw tellt me I came in the nurse's black bag," piped up another urchin.

The lady I was attending was expecting her fourth baby. The midwife on duty arrived a bit later but the baby was in no hurry to make his entry into the world. We sat and ate crusty bread that this busy woman had baked the day before. It was six o'clock at night before the baby was born. We drank endless cups of tea, necessitating trips down the stairs to the communal toilet. After the birth, the husband arrived and insisted we had a dram of Irish whiskey to wet the baby's head. I, at the age of twenty-two had very seldom tasted spirits, so a neat dram of this stuff had me floating along the pavement on my way back home. Definitely a day to remember! The baby was lovely too!

Another confinement I recall on the district was a baby born with the membranes of the placenta over his face.

"Whatever's that over its face?" I whispered, not wanting to alarm the mother. "I've never seen anything like that before."

"It's all right, it's only the membranes covering the face. The baby is fine – it doesn't impede breathing," the midwife reassured me. She showed me how to remove the membranes and a beautiful little boy was uncovered.

"This is known as the caul; in seafaring communities babies born like this are considered to be safe from drowning. Your baby is going to have a lucky life," the midwife assured the mother once the baby was safely delivered.

"My grandad came from the fishing village of Portmahomack, away up north. He would be pleased to know his great grandson's a lucky baby," the delighted mother replied.

"When I visit my boyfriend's home in Lossiemouth, I can see the lighthouse at Portmahomack flashing across the Moray Firth. I'll remember you and your baby now whenever I have a walk along the Lossie beach," I told her.

I enjoyed my eight weeks on the district. I delivered babies and also went on post-natal visits. Mostly the family was in a one or two roomed flat. The new little baby was in a drawer in front of the coal fire that burnt in the grate day and night, the next one up would be wearing a soaking wet terry nappy and a tattered vest, a bottle would be hanging from his mouth. He would generously give the baby a wee suck when it cried. There would be a three-year old jumping over the battered sofa, and the mother would have no help from the father whether he was at home or not. You washed your hands at the cold tap at the box sink set beneath the window, examined the mother's abdomen to make sure the uterus was staying contracted, asked about the colour of her postnatal discharge, to ensure that there was no internal infection. You took her blood pressure and weighed the baby. This was done using an old-fashioned weight and balance. The baby was suspended on a hook, looking for all the world as though it was being brought by the stork. For the first forty-eight hours after a home delivery the mother was visited twice a day, after that it was once a day for ten days.

We had to keep a record of our deliveries in a "blue book" which was used in the final examination A record would read like this:

Mrs Kathleen Smith –Age 18, Para 0 (which meant it was her first
pregnancy)
Last menstrual period or LMP: 22/9/63
Expected date of delivery or EDD: 29/6/64
   12.40am: *Contractions fairly strong – 3-4mins*
   4am: *Contractions fairly strong – 2-3mins. Given Pethidine*
   100mgms intramuscularly
   5.45am: *Fully dilated*
   6.50am: *Normal delivery of a live female child. Syntometrine*
   1mg given with anterior shoulder
1st Stage: 12hours 20mins; 2nd Stage: 50 mins; 3rd Stage: 5 mins.
Blood loss 4oz: Placenta and membranes complete
Infant: Female: Birth weight 7lb 13ozs
Cried after mucus extraction.

And that was the whole drama of birth summed up with abbreviations and jargon, but for the young parents life would never be the same again.

We sat a further examination after the year was over, and this, together with the on-going record of all the deliveries we'd assisted at, gave us the qualification of State Certified Midwife. I passed the examination but by then I had decided I definitely preferred general nursing to midwifery.

"I'm going back to the Royal, Sally," I said. "I've been accepted to work as a senior staff nurse in ward 39. I'm so pleased because female surgical has always been my favourite. What are you planning to do?"

"I'm going to stay on here as a staff midwife for six months, and then I think I'll be moving to Lewis. Roddy's going back to his home territory."

"So obviously you want to be there too," I finished for her. "Good luck, then Sally. We've had a good time together, and you've certainly helped me when I was feeling low."

So I moved back to general nursing, never thinking it would be twenty years before we met again.

Chapter 8: Staff Nurse

The year was 1965. I went back to Glasgow Royal Infirmary and started to work as a senior staff nurse in a female surgical ward. Four and a half years had passed since I was a young trainee and both nursing and I had advanced. There were now far more disposable items of equipment, although we still made up dressings packs and washed and boiled and polished instruments.

As staff nurses we polished our blue and silver hospital badges along with the forceps. We valued these tokens of our achievement as much as when we had been presented with them when we passed our finals to become registered general nurses. The staff nurses' uniform was the smartest I've ever had. We wore dark navy and white striped dresses, the hemline brushing the calves of our legs in the days when the length of our ordinary skirts was moving ever upwards. We still had the inevitable starched collar and cuffs, but our pride and joy was a black belt over the starched apron that all nurses wore. The belt signified that we were senior staff nurses. Dressed like this you felt you could conquer the world, which was just as well, because all sorts of emergencies, sick and acutely ill folk were admitted on a receiving day, crying out "Nurse, nurse, I need a nurse!"

During that year nurses' hours of work were reduced to forty instead of forty-two. This meant you had a half-day a week, so now it was possible to have a half-day on Friday, a day off on Saturday for one week, then a day off on Sunday for the next week, and a morning off on Monday. It meant you could go away for a weekend occasionally, which had never happened before.

Carol was the only one of my crowd who came back with me.

"Sally's going to Stornoway to work because Roddy is being transferred back to his home town," I told Carol, who prophesied, "I should think there'll be wedding bells there soon, lucky her!"

"How's your romance with Bob?" I added. "We've got a year's gossip to catch up on!"

"Oh, it's all off. I'm finished with men, Margaret. I'm going to be a career woman."

"I don't believe that for one minute. The men all fall over each other to ask you out for a date. I'll give you three months at the most!"

"OK. I'll prove you wrong though," Carol said.

"Have you heard from Joan at all?" I asked.

"I met her in Copland's before I came back to staff here," she replied. "Her romance with Kenny has cooled off a bit. She's still in Edinburgh, staffing at the Simpson's."

"It must be so difficult for them to meet regularly, what with her shifts and his hours. I find it bad enough to find time to go out with David. He's studying for his finals, and I'm often on a late shift on Saturday. At least we don't get bored with one another's company!"

If we had an afternoon off on the same day, Carol and I used to go into town together and browse round the shops. Now we were staff nurses we had a bit more money to spend on clothes and make up and anyway we could always window shop, especially in the Argyle Arcade, Glasgow's one and only covered shopping mall where jewellery shops displayed sparkling engagement rings.

"Being a man free zone hasn't spoiled your enjoyment at looking at engagement rings, Carol," I teased her. "We're both experts in the field."

"Well, there's no harm in keeping up to date with the latest styles is there," she replied.

Sometimes we went into the staff nurses' sitting room and spent our afternoon off dozing in ancient armchairs reeking with stale cigarette smoke.

"It's a right fug in here, Carol," I said. "I'm going for a cup of tea before we go back on duty. How are you enjoying your ward? I'm loving staffing in female surgical. I like Heather so much, she's the best sister I've ever worked with."

Heather was young, proactive and always pleasant.

"I like a Thursday evening off because it's my badminton night. I hope you don't mind working regularly that night, Margaret. Don't worry, I'll try to give you time off when you want as well."

I nearly fell over backwards in surprise. A sister, asking me about her off duty? I knew that life was going to be much easier for me now.

Heather worked along with the nurses, giving out bedpans and feeding patients. She also made time for patients' relatives, advising them how the patient was progressing, if the wound was healing, when the stitches were due to come out, when the patient was likely to go home. She encouraged me to do the same, and I thought that was a much better arrangement, rather than sitting in the office expecting worried folk to come and seek us out.

Heather called her staff by their Christian names, and was glad for the staff nurses to do the same to her. This familiarity didn't mean there was a lowering of standards of care.

Wound care in particular was meticulously carried out. Using the knowledge of the day, we enthusiastically irrigated, drained and packed wounds, and horror of horrors by today's reasoning, we shaved the skin before surgery. An irate surgeon might summon a nurse into theatre to remove a hair that had escaped a blunt razor blade. The humiliation of that prospect ensured skin as bare as a baby's bottom!

"Great news," Carol greeted me in the changing room before we went on duty. "Joan's romance is on again and she's going to be married. I had a letter from her."

"Oh, fantastic," I said. "She's the first one of us to get hitched. The last I heard of Sally, she hadn't finalised her wedding plans, though she's moved up to Stornoway. When's the happy day?"

"Next March," said Carol. "And I think we'll be invited to the wedding."

"Even more fantastic," I replied. "Oh, gosh, it's nearly ten to eight, we'll have to get our skates on to be on duty in time."

So we rushed along the corridors and up the stairs, my ward was on the fifth floor and Carol's was on the fourth.

The stairs didn't stop our tongues from moving as fast as our feet. We talked about this latest piece of news all the way, discussing what Joan's dress would be like, and what we could find in our wardrobes for ourselves to wear.

However when I arrived at the ward I forgot about the wedding in the rush of work. At that time surgeons in my unit were beginning to operate on patients with vascular disease. Heather reported, "There's a lady called Mrs Dunlop coming in this afternoon for a bypass graft. We'll prepare the single bedded cubicle as an intensive care unit. Mrs Dunlop will be given special individual nursing care for four days postoperatively. You and I and Jeanette the most senior student will be the ones to look after her, checking her vital signs and monitoring her condition every fifteen minutes until she is stabilised."

This was pioneering work. I had never nursed anyone after this kind of surgery. I was staggered at the number of tubes and drips I had to monitor when Mrs Dunlop returned from theatre. She was in our ward for over a month and Heather and I were thrilled to watch her progress after such innovative treatment.

As well as patients like Mrs Dunlop, we nursed the usual mix of general surgical conditions: appendicitis; ulcerative colitis; duodenal ulcers, cancer of the bowel, pancreas and liver. A nineteen-year-old girl called Marie was admitted with severe abdominal pain. It turned out that Marie had an ectopic pregnancy and because she was unmarried, confessing to being pregnant was difficult for her. Unmarried mothers were sent to mother and baby homes where the baby was taken away for adoption at birth. The surgeon on duty probed the true facts from her with gentleness and sensitivity. I don't know if she realised that he saved her life by his experience in palpating her tender, tense abdomen.

As I accompanied the senior consultants on the ward round I was very impressed by their knowledge and skill. These eminent surgeons relied on the techniques they'd learnt over many years in their everyday judgement of the patient's condition.

Another young woman on the ward had been admitted with severe ulcerated colitis and the surgeons had to remove a large portion of her bowel.

"I'm really worried about Sadie," I reported to Heather. "The ileostomy bag keeps leaking. All that liquid faeces are pouring out over her wound and it's horribly infected. Her skin is so sore it's like a lump of raw of meat. She's in agony."

"I know. She's so young and she only got married last year. It's bad enough having an ileostomy, she doesn't need all the trauma of a gaping wound and excoriated skin as well," Heather said. "Let's keep on with the savlon baths twice a day and put on plenty of barrier cream around the stoma."

Sadie was in the ward for weeks. When she went home at last we felt we were losing a friend. During her long ordeal she had never complained, and had encouraged other women as they went to theatre. We were sad to wave goodbye but we were all thankful she had made a good recovery.

Another lady who was in and out of the ward was Jeannie. Jeannie had suffered from rheumatic heart disease when she was a child. Several pregnancies had weakened her heart. She was also a heavy smoker and was admitted with gangrene of her right leg.

Her only hope was to have vascular surgery. Unfortunately it was unsuccessful, so Jeannie had to have more surgery: her right leg was amputated below the knee. The stump refused to heal, so she then had an above knee amputation. In spite of all this, Jeannie made a good recovery and went home. She was a cheery soul who never complained, despite all she suffered. Three months later, Heather said, "I'm afraid Jeannie is to be readmitted today. Her left leg has become gangrenous now. It will be have to be amputated too "

"Poor Jeannie! We really thought she was better. I hate to think she's got to lose her other leg. I'll go and make up a bed for her right now," I said

Without her legs Jeannie was as light as a feather. I carried her in my arms so that she could chat to her friends at the top of the ward. But then Jeannie had a stroke. She was too ill to be taken to a medical ward and so we nursed her until she died. She was in her early fifties, and left a husband who was devoted to her, and whom we'd got to know really well, he'd been a faithful visitor all this time.

As well as these patients we had our usual quota of old ladies with fractured femurs. One old lady was so fond of her husband, and he was of her.

"Davie James," she called out to him. "Davie James, I miss you, Davie James, you should be here by now! Where are you Davie James?"

Then one day she became very confused, so often the outcome after the shock of the fall, and the anaesthetic; she didn't know him when he visited. He bought her orchids, a great rarity, but she tried to tear them up.

"Take these weeds away!" she shouted.

We put them at the end of the ward out of her sight. That weekend was Joan's wedding.

"Would you like one of these orchids, Margaret? It would make an exotic corsage for your outfit," Heather said. "It's a shame to keep such expensive flowers hidden away in a corner."

"Are you sure? I've never worn an orchid before. Thanks very much, Heather. See you on Sunday."

Joan looked gorgeous in her wedding dress, which was straight and high necked, showing her slender figure.

"We always knew Joan would make a beautiful bride," Carol told me. "And that's a great outfit you're wearing, Margaret," she added.

I'd borrowed my sister's canary yellow dress, a Mary Quant design with a daring hemline. Mini skirts were just coming into fashion. I looked and felt good in the new smart style. David was very appreciative too!

"I love you in that new look, Margaret," he said. "Is that really an orchid you're wearing?"

I had a fleeting vision of Davie James and his rejected gift.

Sunday morning and a busy day shift came far too soon. We had a new admission, another fractured femur. This patient, in her early sixties, had fallen at home. After admission she became extremely aggressive and we realised that she was an alcoholic, suffering from withdrawal symptoms.

"I thought alcoholics are old dossers drinking Brasso or hair lacquer," I said to Heather, "But this lady doesn't seem like that at all. She's so well spoken and I saw when I admitted her that she comes from Langside. That's quite a posh area, isn't it?"

"Things aren't always as they seem," said Heather. "Net curtains can hide a lot."

Years later when I became a district nurse I often remembered those words. She never said a truer thing!

There were patients in the ward with breast cancer. They went to theatre for a biopsy. Tissue was sent to the laboratory whilst the patient was still under the anaesthetic. If the tumour proved to be malignant, the breast was removed. Still groggy from the anaesthetic the women would immediately put their hands up to their breast to see if it was still there. If there were bulky dressings and drains in place, they knew the breast had been removed.

The work in our surgical ward was demanding. Heather was very dedicated and always worked way past her time for going off duty. We were a good team of sister, staff and student nurses, together with the junior hospital doctors who spent six months in a surgical ward and six months in a medical the first year after they qualified. The change over period was in August and February.

"Oh, no, it's the residents' change over time again. We'll have to teach another new one how to do all the procedures here the way our surgeons want things done," Heather and I said to each other.

The junior doctors were thrown in at the deep end and were glad of any help that nurses could give them. Our new resident was Helen. This was the first time I'd worked with a young female doctor, a sign that more women were entering the medical profession.

"I don't know how you keep going with so little sleep, Helen. I know you've been up out of your bed the last forty-eight hours," I said to her when we were wheeling a trolley up the ward for her to set up a blood transfusion.

"It's a tough year," she admitted. "I'm so tired all the time, I'm terrified I'll prescribe the wrong dose of a drug, especially when I have to calculate the amount in my head."

"No, it's not safe being on call day and night," I agreed. "You need a proper night shift Can't you complain to the senior doctors? "

"Medicine is still male dominated, and the old school tie reigns supreme," Helen answered. "The attitude is 'if it was good enough for me it is good enough for you.' We want a job after the year's up so we just keep going."

To help these overworked doctors, we filled in various forms and certificates so all they had to do was sign them. I also made out lists of jobs for the nurses, so that the nursing care was done as prescribed by Heather and me. The nurses knew exactly what they had to do, the patients appreciated our care and the well-run ward had a happy atmosphere, conducive to healing.

Outside nursing changes were on the horizon for me. David and I were planning our wedding. Now I was one of the nurses who put on my engagement ring in the dining room for my friends to admire. We carried our rings in their boxes in our pockets so that they were handy to put on at every opportunity. For years I had admired other people's rings, now I was showing off my own. But we didn't think we were showing off, it was the done thing. We were all experts in different types of rings. "Susie's got three in a straight, Maggie's got three in a twist, Jane's got a cluster." This had been the talk at the meal table for years, when we hadn't been talking shop!

"Are you going to stay on after you're married, Margaret?" Carol asked.

"No, we've got a flat near the University. I'm applying for a part time staff nurse's post in the Western Infirmary. Guess what, Joan's working in the Western now. I bumped into her in Dumbarton Road. I'd been over to look at our new flat. She and Kenny actually live in the next street. What about you, Carol, are you planning to move on?"

"I've been accepted for the sister's post in a male surgical ward," Carol informed me.

"That's tremendous news. You'll be a very good ward sister."

"Well, I hope so. It's what we've been trained for, isn't it?

So I left the ward I'd been so happy in. I'd learned a lot and grown up a lot. I'd coped with responsibility and looked after ill and dying patients, consoled grieving relatives, and seen suffering and loss borne with courage, humour and endurance. Glasgow folk will always be high in my estimation!

Chapter 9: All Change

I left the Royal Infirmary and said goodbye to my patients in Ward 39 in June 1966. Two weeks later the sun shone on my wedding day. My friends all came to my wedding, but it was three months later before Carol and I managed to meet in town for a cup of coffee.

"How's it going being a sister?" I asked.

"Oh, it's great. I'm enjoying it very much. We're very busy, but it's good doing things the way I want. I'm trying to cut out some of the paper work. Nurses shouldn't have to waste time on secretarial stuff... I've got a new love in my life, and this time I'm sure it's for real," Carol went on.

"Oh, good, who's the lucky lad?" I said, pleased that things were going well for Carol in her personal as well as her professional life.

"His name's Peter, he's a P.E teacher. What about you, Margaret? Have you started that part-time job yet?"

"Well, no, I think I'll be doing the practical side of midwifery."

"Oh, gosh! You're not pregnant already. How far on are you?"

"I'm about fourteen weeks, so I haven't thought about work. It's a bit of a shock so soon after our wedding."

"I should think so, but these things happen! But, Margaret, are you sure you're all right? You don't look very well. You're terribly pale. Are you really OK?"

"I'm fine. I had morning sickness, but it's worn off thank goodness. But strangely, I've just started feeling dizzy. I'd better go home."

"Yes, you do that. Take care, Margaret. Go and lie down for a bit."

"I'll see you later, Carol. Cheerio."

So I went home, but in fact I was having a miscarriage. I was taken to the Western Infirmary for surgery. I was in hospital for four days – so now I was experiencing life as a patient, but although I received good care I was shocked at losing my first baby.

Carol and Joan both visited me in the hospital with gifts of flowers and my favourite talc and scent.

"You've been a great help to me," I said, as we met in my flat one evening, a couple of weeks after my operation. "I think I feel ready to go back to work now."

"It's the best thing for you to do!" They were unanimous in their opinion.

"What's it like nursing in the Western?" I asked Joan. "I've only been a patient!"

"It's OK, but as a part time staff nurse, they call you 'Mrs', not 'Nurse'."

"That's making us like second-class citizens!" I protested, "Well too bad! I'm going to be working thirty four hours a week."

"I do thirty six," Joan said. "I'm in male surgical. The uniform is nice, but the dresses have long sleeves and starched cuffs. It's a right carry on with those cuffs. You take them off and roll up your sleeves when you're with the patients. If you're doing a doctors' round, you have to pull the sleeves down, button up all the wee footery buttons and put on the cuffs. Half the time you forget where you left them and grab somebody else's," she told me.

"Thanks for telling me. I wonder which ward they'll put me in?"

I walked home with Joan one evening the following week.

"How're you doing, Margaret?"

"Oh, Joan, you'll never guess. I'm in Gynae. The very same ward I was in a month ago as a patient. The first person I met was the resident. 'Haven't I seen you before, your face looks familiar,' he said. Well, Joan, I nearly died. I felt like telling him it was actually not my face he'd seen. He'd been in theatre when I had my D and C."

"How embarrassing. Of all the wards to be sent to!"

"I know. It's not easy at all. The girl who was in the next bed to me is still there. She's had several miscarriages, so she has to stay in hospital to try to stop her losing her baby. I thought it was bad enough having one miscarriage! The good thing is, I know exactly what she's going through but I feel a bit emotional when I've just lost my baby. I've always liked Gynae, but do you know, Joan, I dread going there every day."

"I'm sure you do. Perhaps you should ask for a transfer."

In fact, a few weeks later I was moved to the Eye Department.

"Eyes," I said to Joan. "I know absolutely nothing about eyes."

"Never mind, you'll learn a lot. The Eye Department is a prestigious institute," she told me

Being part time, my work was mainly in the clinic. It seemed far too tame after the drama of the busy ward I'd worked in as a full time staff nurse. However, there was a ward upstairs so I could still give actual nursing care to patients.

The other staff nurse in the clinic was older, maybe as much as fifty, which seemed ancient to my twenty-four years! Her name was Hughina McCuish, and she came from Lewis.

"I've never been to Lewis – or to any of the Hebrides except a day trip to Iona once," I said, "but I have a friend there called Sally, she's just got married to a Lewisman, Roddy MacDonald. They're both in Stornoway, he's a policeman…"

"Och, Margaret I've known the family for years. I was at the school with his auntie," she replied. "It's a small world indeed."

Hughina showed me round the clinic. We had to call the waiting patients and do a basic sight test. If the patients couldn't see well enough to read the top letter of the chart we held up our fingers for them to count. With young children we used a chart shaped like a letter E and turned it different ways to test their vision.

Calling a patient's name could be fraught with difficulty.

"Miss Bugue," I called out, pronouncing it "Bug."

A highly offended lady marched up to me. "My name is Bugue with a long U," she informed me indignantly.

I learned how to test patients' intra ocular pressure, using a machine with a blue light. We looked into the patients' eyes through the light and the reading was a diagnostic tool for determining if they had glaucoma.

We tested for colour blindness using a book with different colour dots all jumbled together. This was known as the Ishihara test.

Sometimes people had to wait hours in the clinic, especially if they were seeing the professor who taught medical students about the various conditions his patients had. One young couple brought in their little girl with a rare genetic condition that also affected her eyes. The parents had to wait outside his consulting room and I had to hold the severely handicapped child for the students to observe.

"The condition is called 'Cri du Chat'," the professor informed them. "If you know your French, you will know this means the cry of the cat and that is exactly how an infant like this cries."

Just at that moment the wee girl obliged by giving a meowing sound which sounded so like a cat I nearly dropped her in my surprise.

"The syndrome causes severe mental retardation, and a short life expectancy," he went on with clinical detachment. I cuddled the little girl close trying to protect her from the harsh reality of her life.

There was a contact lens clinic run by an optician. Patients whose eyesight was unable to be corrected by spectacles were given contact lenses on the NHS. There were children in that category. Some were extremely short-sighted; others presented with the pale eyes, devoid of pigment, of albinism.

I thought that if they could cope with contact lenses, I would have a go as well. So I took the plunge, made an appointment with an optician and was fitted with contact lenses, thankfully consigning the glasses I'd worn since early childhood to history.

"You look great without your glasses," Joan said.

"Thank you," I said. "I tell you what's wonderful, I can see my feet in the bath! It's fine at the hairdresser's too. I can see what they're doing. Before I would put my glasses on, look in the mirror, and think, 'I don't like what they've done to my hair.' I tell you a new world has opened up for me. It's been one good thing to come out of the Eye Department. There are such sad wee kids there. Just now in the ward we've got two wee boys with retinoblastoma."

"Whatever's that? It sounds awful."

"It's a cancer that affects the retina of one eye. It can be contained, but only by having the affected eye removed and the good eye blasted with radiotherapy."

"Oh, Margaret, how dreadful! I didn't know cancer attacks the eyes. Poor little boys! How old are they?"

"One's eighteen months and the other's three. Wee Jimmy, the wee one of eighteen months is so gorgeous. He's got masses of curls, and just looks a picture. He stands at the end of his cot and yells for his mum when the visiting hour's over. She brings him holy water from Lourdes in a little silver cup. He gets a drink every time she's there."

"Let's hope it helps. I'll light a candle for him when I go to Mass on Sunday."

Joan often told us how her faith helped her to deal with all the tragedies we'd come across in our nursing careers.

"That's lovely. I'm sure she'd be pleased to know that. I pray for my patients too," I said.

"Yes, I know you do, remember we sometimes went to those morning prayers in the hospital chapel in the Royal? Prayer's a strange thing, isn't it?"

"We've got a man in who believes in good luck rather than prayer," I said. "He says he's the seventh child of the seventh child. He tells us he has the second sight. He was admitted blind in both eyes, but he had a corneal graft so now he can see a bit."

"It's marvellous that he can see again," Joan said.

"Yes, he's over the moon. He peers into the tea cups to read people's fortunes. The patients in the ward queue up with their empty cups to get their tea leaves read. You should hear the stories he tells. Second sight is all very well, he says, but he's so pleased now he's got even a glimmer of the real thing."

"Modern medicine is improving so many folks' lives," Joan commented.

Laser treatment was being pioneered in the department. Three brothers came by train from Dorset in the south of England. They were in their thirties, and each one was going blind as a result of diabetic retinopathy. The laser treatment was their only hope.

Laser treatment was also used for a little girl of six from Ayrshire. Janie had a birthmark at the back of her eye, known as a haemangioma. She had five younger brothers and sisters. Her parents hardly ever came to visit although she was in the ward for weeks. The ward sister took her under her wing and let her sit at the desk whilst she wrote the report. Janie loved the sister. She was a very glamorous lady, with long glossy black hair she wore parted in the middle and piled high up on her head. Her name was Chrissie Anne Macleod, and she came from Harris. She used to kid people on, saying that the initials C.A on her badge stood for Conchita Anita. With her dark Spanish looks and Highland accent they really believed her.

Patients in the eye ward were admitted for surgery for cataracts and detached retinas. They had to lie in bed for a long time after surgery with both eyes bandaged and had to be washed and fed. They were forbidden to reach over to their lockers even for a drink. It must have been extremely boring for them, especially as they were fit and well otherwise.

One lady came from North Uist to have her cataracts removed. Old Mrs McIver, eighty-eight years old had both her eyes done at the same time. Hughina came up from the clinic occasionally to speak to her in Gaelic, and Sister MacLeod was able to talk to her in her own language too.

The day she was going home, Mrs McIver was up early to be ready for her flight on the small Logan Air aeroplane. She slipped in the bathroom and fractured her femur. She had to be transferred to an orthopaedic ward. I don't know if she ever went back to her island home.

One evening in early spring Carol and Joan came round to my flat.

"I've got news for you," Carol said. "Peter got that job he applied for, teaching PE in high school in Montreal. We'll be going off in August, right after our wedding."

"Shall I tell you something?" Joan said. "We're going to Canada too."

"Never!" we exclaimed together.

"Yes, Kenny's going to be a consultant in Toronto. He's to start in June. I'm thrilled to bits but I'm sorry to be missing your wedding, Carol."

"Well, I hope I'll be able to come to your big day," I said. "I've got news too. I'm expecting a baby. It's due in September."

"Oh, that's great news – and you look so well this time, I'm sure everything will be okay for you. You'd better not dance an Eightsome Reel at the wedding reception," Carol said. "I'll be wearing a wedding dress, not a midwife's gown; we don't want a delivery on the dance floor."

We all laughed. "The band would have a fit," Joan said.

"So would David! I tell you something, it's maybe a good thing I'm working in the clinic after all. I don't do any heavy lifting."

I hoped so much that this time nothing would go wrong and I would have a lovely baby.

And so it proved. I left work in the summer time and went to Carol's wedding. I didn't dance the Eightsome Reel, but just the same a few days later I gave birth to a beautiful baby boy. My nursing career was put on hold for a while.

Chapter 10: Pastures New

The year was 1973. I was now the mother of two little boys; we lived in Aberdeen. I felt the time had come to try to return to nursing. David had a job that took him away from home, therefore I decided to work as a relief nurse.

"That's the good thing about nursing nowadays," I said to David. "It's possible to work hours that suit married women. Times have certainly changed even since we were married, and my part time hours were thirty-four a week."

The local general hospital was also a teaching hospital, of which the people of Aberdeen were proud. When the present building was erected in the nineteen thirties the money was raised by voluntary subscription, and workers had so much a week deducted from their wages, so Aberdonians felt their hospital truly belonged to them.

Changes had occurred in the five years I had been away from hospital life. On average, the patients were older. Better anaesthetic drugs and more antibiotics meant that extensive surgery was now possible, while in the medical wards especially, the drug trolley contained medicine I had never heard of.

I was often sent to the neurosurgery unit. I felt quite apprehensive at first. I had never worked in this speciality before. Now I was caring for patients recovering from brain surgery. They all required intensive monitoring. I learnt about the Glasgow Coma Scale used to determine whether the patient was regaining consciousness or slipping deeper into a coma. Some of the patients would reach a level of consciousness where they became very confused and aggressive, trying to pull out their tubes and get out of bed.

I often worked with another part-time staff nurse called Janet, country born and bred, like so many nurses in Aberdeen. "D'ye mind on Robert?" Janet asked me one night, as we were putting on the staff nurses' uniform, pale red dresses, which gave us the nickname of 'Pinkie'.

"Isn't he that fourteen-year-old boy who lost his whole family in that terrible road accident? Remember their car was behind a timber lorry; some logs came loose and crushed them all? Robert still didn't know anything about it last time I was on duty. He was deeply unconscious."

"He's come roon' a good bittie. His recordings were all fine and stable, so maybe he's on the road to recovery."

Happily Robert continued to improve and went home to be cared for by his grandparents.

You read of road accidents in the news and see crashed cars on television but it's easy to forget the reality of the lasting damage the patients are left with. I was brought face to face with it every night I worked in this unit, hoping that the care given by the neurosurgery team, doctors, nurses and physiotherapists would restore our patients to some degree of normal ability.

Aberdeen hospitals serve the community of Banff and Buchan, the heartland of Doric speech, and also patients from Orkney and Shetland come down from their island homes for specialist care.

Many of the staff, both doctors and nurses, also belonged to this area, especially then, just before the coming of North Sea oil changed the population of Aberdeen to a more cosmopolitan one. Doctors, nurses and patients alike still spoke Broad Scots. Being married to a man from Lossiemouth, I found that the Doric of the Aberdeenshire folk was a bit different from the speech of the Moray Firth fishing communities. I sometimes had problems understanding some of the old folk, especially if they had no teeth! If you don't come from the North East of Scotland, you too would find it difficult to understand a cry of distress like this, " I'm affa sorry Nursie, but I was haeing my fly cuppie, and I coupit it ower and teemed it on the flair."

I wasn't alone. Flora came from a little Highland village and had never heard the North East speech until she trained in Aberdeen in the

1950s. She worked in the Sick Children's Hospital. A dragon of a ward sister, annoyed because Flora was taking so long to feed the very sick babies, marched her into a room with a large, highly polished table, and ordered her to "Redd oot this place and get rid of all the stew." Flora had looked around her baffled. "This place must be used for meetings, what with that grand table and all those portraits of severe looking doctors," she had thought. "Why would there be a pot of stew here?"

However, she obediently polished the table so that it gleamed even more, wondering all the time where on earth the stew was and what would she do with it if she found any. It was long after before she discovered that stew is the Scots word for dust!

Life as a relief staff nurse was very varied. I was sent to a different ward almost every week. We were often too busy to go for meal breaks and so we would try to snatch an illicit cup of coffee before waking the patients in the morning. Once, when I was in the respiratory unit, where a lot of patients were on oxygen I started to make toast for me and the student nurse, Anne. Unfortunately while my back was turned the toast stuck in the toaster. Flames shot out of the top and Anne came rushing back in.

"It's OK, it's burning itself out! " I said, trying to stay calm. We both breathed a sigh of relief. "All this oxygen in the atmosphere! We could have burnt the place down, imagine trying to evacuate patients strung up to all those tubes and machines."

That morning in particular I was glad to be able to report in the nursing Kardex my patients had a "Good night, slept well."

This was the usual comment, but one that was often denied by the patient in the morning.

"I havena closed my e'en the hale nicht" they would say, but they'd been snoring peacefully each time I'd passed the bed.

One source of disturbance was caused by oystercatchers. These birds mistook the flat roof of the hospital for cliff tops, and nested there. In the early mornings of summer, when it is hardly dark at all in the north east of Scotland, they piped their shrill cries from two a.m. Then there was justification for the patients' complaint of sleeplessness! In spite of this inconvenience, the patients and nurses enjoyed watching the birds on their nests, and we followed the progress of the chicks when they hatched out.

Working in Aberdeen was the first time I looked after patients who had spinal injuries. A good-looking young lad called Ian, on leave from the army, had been helping out on his parents' farm. A fall had left him totally paralysed from the neck down. Ian was distraught and extremely depressed. He was in the ward for months and I was sad to watch him give up the unequal struggle to survive. His breathing became shallow as hope faded from his eyes.

One night I went into the ward and saw in the report, "Ian Smith had a respiratory arrest at 3.25p.m. Resuscitation was unsuccessful."

Another patient who, like Ian was totally paralysed, was a fisherman called Dod Campbell. He had fallen down the hold of his fishing vessel. Dod eventually got back a very slight degree of movement in his right hand. You would have thought he'd won the football pools, he was so thrilled!

"I'm coming on just great, I'll be awa' to the dancing the morn," he told us with a smile although he knew very well that he would never gain any more mobility. He knew too that he would never regain an independent life, but he didn't let that get him down. One day he told me the good news that he was going to be transferred to a small hospital in the fishing village a couple of miles from his home.

"It's fine to be going hame. A' my freens'll be in to see me. It'll be much less of a trauchle for the wife as weel. She's gey weary wi' this aye traipsing back and fore. I canna thank you quines enough for whit ye've a' deen for me."

Sometimes there were pictures of him in the local paper, strapped in his wheelchair, in full evening dress attending a wedding or a fisherman's dinner, so we knew he was still keeping his spirits up. Dod was truly one of life's great unsung heroes.

Another great character was a confused old lady called Sophie. She was always trying to do the nurses a good turn.

One night old Sophie thought she was helping us by gathering in little plastic pots with lids from the patients' lockers. She was up wandering at three a.m, when I was busy with a lady who had undergone major chest surgery. I needed to be in and out of her single room frequently during the night. I came out of her open door to see a night-gowned figure disappearing into one of the other rooms along the corridor.

I hurried along the ward to see what was happening. There was Sophie with her hands full of little blue pots.

"Aye, Nursie, I've scored oot a' these dishes for you. I've been fairly kept at it the hale nicht. Noo I'm awa' tae hae a lookie in here. I'll maybe find some mair tae dee."

"Oh, Sophie, that's all the false teeth from the patients' lockers you've got," I exclaimed, caught between laughter and exasperation. "I don't know how I'll ever get them all back to the right folk. You go away to your bed and have a sleep. You shouldn't be up wandering around at this time of night."

I helped the old lady back to bed. Old Sophie was too confused to notice my dismay – after all, she'd only been doing an act of kindness!

By now, oil had been discovered in the North Sea. Workers in the oil industry sometimes had serious accidents. I looked after Klaus, a German lad who had suffered severe injuries. His job was to dig trenches for the pipeline bringing gas from the oil rigs. A digger sliced through him whilst he was working in the trench, mutilating him terribly. Klaus had to have both a colostomy and urostomy and he wore two drainage bags attached to the stomas on either side of his abdomen. Klaus had several operations for reconstruction of his genital and internal organs and eventually went home to Germany for hospital treatment there.

Some patients were flown to the hospital landing strip by helicopter. The disaster on the Piper Alpha oil platform saw helicopters taking off and landing all night although, tragically, so many men had perished out at sea that most of the helicopters returned empty.

Surgery was advancing all the time. Kidney transplants were being performed successfully, coronary artery bypass operations were now the norm rather than pioneering work, and patients were being discharged home more quickly than had been the case ten years previously.

I gave continual nursing care to John, a twenty-year-old from Orkney, brain damaged in a diving accident. He had been diving at Scapa Flow and surfaced too quickly. He was flown to Aberdeen for treatment in the Hyperbaric Unit, a decompression chamber used to treat divers for the condition known as 'the bends'. Unfortunately John was left permanently handicapped despite the latest technology. His father came down from Orkney to sit with him. I was glad to talk to his father about Orkney. Perhaps his anxiety was relieved for a while as we travelled in our minds across the sea to the green fertile islands in the north.

As my boys grew older, I worked during the day rather than at night. The hours suited my family commitments – I was now looking after my mother in the advanced stages of Parkinson's Disease.

Other changes had happened for my friends too. Carol was now home from Canada and we often chatted on the phone.

"How are you settling in Montrose? David and I are so pleased that you're back in Scotland. I'm dying to see you all."

"You'll have to come and visit," Carol invited. "The kids are getting bigger, Susie's nine and Grant is six. Peter's enjoying his new job, but it'll be some time before I get back to nursing. How are you doing?"

"It's fine being a relief nurse from the point of view of suitable working hours, but I don't really feel part of the ward team because you get moved all the time. The permanent staff nurses half my age are sitting at the desk writing reports and giving orders while I'm rushing about doing the work."

"I know what you mean," Carol said, "After all, we're both nearly forty now – what a thought. How do you cope with it all, especially looking after your mother as well? How is she now?"

"A district nurse comes in to help me bath her. It's a great help and it's a support emotionally too."

Not long after this conversation my mother died at home in my house. I was very impressed with the care given to her day and night by nurses from the District Nursing service.

Soon after my mother's death I got a phone call asking me to go out into the community to help district nurses who were short staffed as a flu virus raged in Aberdeen.

I so enjoyed nursing people at home in their own environment. The years fell away. I remembered visiting Mrs Docherty at home and the women and babies I'd cared for on the district in my midwifery training.

Now I learned about the District Nursing Course held in the Nursing College in the same complex as the hospital. I was accepted on to the eight-month course, so after a gap of twenty-two years, I became a student once more.

Chapter 11: Back to College

It was now 1982, and I became a mature student on a post-registration course in a college of nursing. The minimum professional requirement for entry to the course was to be a registered general nurse with two years staff nurse experience. The other essential requirement was a driving licence. The days of district nurses cycling on their rounds was over, although as the traffic density worsened, a bicycle sometimes seemed a good idea...But not in driving rain and gales of wind screaming in off the North Sea!

The students came from all over the North of Scotland. I made friends with Sheila, a twenty-four-year old staff nurse. Sheila was a country girl, brought up on a farm in a remote part of Aberdeenshire.

"When I finished my training I went awa up to Shetland to work in the Gilbert Bain hospital," Sheila told me. "I wanted a complete change."

"That was definitely different," I agreed. "And quite a big step when you were only twenty-one. Did you like it up there? I've never been to Shetland, but I love going to Orkney, so I can imagine a bit what your life was like."

"I had a great time there and would have liked fine to stay, but efter a year I applied to work in intensive care in Edinburgh. I didna want to get stuck in a rut."

"There's no chance of that with you, Sheila. What an adventurous nursing life you've had!" I said, "And here's you doing the district nursing course now. I'm sure we'll all enjoy this new challenge."

My other friends were married like myself. Chrissie came from Lewis and I told her about my friend Sally.

"We trained in the Royal and did midder together," I told Chrissie. "Sally married a policeman called Roddy MacDonald."

"Och yes, I know fine who you're speaking about. Sally and I worked in Stornoway, but that was before we had our families. Roddy was moved to Shetland, but we still see them when they come to see his mother who's all alone on the croft."

Another island nurse was Molly who had left Yorkshire to start a new life in the Inner Hebrides with her teenage family.

"The island is so beautiful and I love the work. It's a different way of life. Our clinics are timed to fit in with the ferry. The bloods have to go to the hospital on the mainland to be tested, so I have to rush down to the harbour with all the specimens. Some of the tourists would be surprised to discover what's in the parcels they're travelling alongside!"

"It's as well they don't know. They might be seasick if they thought about it," Chrissie added.

"It must be a big change for your kids, Molly," I observed.

"It is, and there are plusses and minuses. Kids have to leave the island when they're twelve. They go to secondary school on the mainland and only come home in the holidays," Molly went on.

"Do they stay in a hostel?" I asked.

"Yes, that's why I could get away to do this course, but I don't like them being boarded out and they're not so happy either. I'll finish this course and see what happens."

"It's a worry having teenage kids. My older boy is into all the trendy gear. One thing I'm pleased about is that he's good at music. He plays in the school brass band," I said.

"You tell him to stick in with that," Molly said. "Coming from Yorkshire, I think brass bands are the best. What instrument does he play?"

"The trombone," I replied. " It's got more uses than you'd think, it's handy for bringing home the things he's made in the cookery class. He filled the bell of the trombone with Cornish pasties last night. They were really tasty but when he practised in the evening a strong scent of onions wafted out!"

The course consisted of study in college and experience in the community with a district nurse who had a second qualification as a practical work teacher.

We learned about the history of district nursing. William Rathbone, a nineteenth century philanthropist in Liverpool saw how important home nursing was after his wife had died of cancer. He had employed nurses to work in his home and used his wealth to fund a community nursing service. We also studied social policy, sociology, psychology and theories of learning. As a result, I realised that while my previous training had taught me to cope with anything I met in nursing I had not been taught to think analytically.

At last the time came to go out in the community for practical experience. For Chrissie and Molly this meant a return to the work and homes they'd left behind.

"I'm so glad to be going back to my own fireside," Chrissie said with relief. "I can't get used to living in digs at all. It'll be so fine to see my family again."

I had already been introduced to Liz, my practical work teacher and now, my first day on the district we met in the car park.

"We'll work together for the first couple of weeks," Liz explained, as she started her Mini. "As you know, my role is to assess your practical skills, not because you're not experienced but because there's s big difference between working in the hospital and in a patient's home. The first thing to remember," she continued, "is that the patient doesn't sign a consent form for treatment. The nurse is a guest in the house and if the patient refuses care, then that's their right. That's quite a difficult thing to cope with if you see somebody who is really in need of care."

"So what can you do about it?" I asked.

"You can find ways round most things if you try. Sometimes it can take a while to gain a patient's trust. You often find that these are the very ones who come to rely on you so much that it's hard to take them off the books."

Our first patient was new to Liz too.

"Mr Anderson discharged himself from hospital after surgery for cancer of the larynx," Liz told me. "He lives with his wife in a high rise flat. He should have learnt in the hospital how to care for his laryngeal tube, but he didn't stay in long enough. We've got a real challenge ahead of us to gain his co-operation and help him get used to having no speech."

"How's his wife managing?" I asked. "She must be in a fair old state, I'm sure I would be. Imagine dealing with your husband's tracheostomy, and him not able to speak to you."

"I'm glad you thought about her," Liz said, "because it will be crucial for us to include Mrs Anderson. She's the one who has to cope twenty-four hours a day. Once we've been going to him a few days, I'll let you take over his care. You have to have a caseload of your own, but don't worry, I'll still be around to help."

We discovered from the medical notes that Mr Anderson had developed syphilis when he was a soldier in the Second World War.

"In my student nurse training, I learned about the dilemma doctors had, whether to use penicillin to treat the men with VD and get them back to their regiments or to give it to soldiers with wound infections," I recalled. "The doctor who gave us the lectures explained that penicillin was such a new drug there wasn't enough to go round. Although the Army doctors treated the men with syphilis they didn't give them enough penicillin to prevent them going on to the tertiary stage later in life. Rationing care is definitely not a new concept."

"You're a walking encyclopaedia, Margaret," Liz replied with a laugh.

So in Aberdeen in the nineteen eighties we saw a man with the symptoms of syphilis, the strange gait and the aggression that were part of the end stages of the disease.

"We'll visit him every day, twice a day to begin with, " Liz said. "It will help Mrs Anderson too."

Mrs Anderson and I learned together to teach her uncooperative husband how to care for his 'trachie' tube, and how gradually to go without the tube as his stoma healed.

"You've fairly got on well there, Margaret," Liz said one day after she had made her usual weekly visit. "They'll miss you when you go back to the college."

"I'll miss them too," I said. "I'm finding it easier to communicate with Mr Anderson now".

I discovered some of Liz's patients were not so happy with a new nurse.

"Faur's oor Lizzie the day, she's nae been tae see me a' wik. It's nae eese at a'." Mr Jack complained to me.

"It's OK, Mr Jack, she's not forgotten you, " I reassured him. "I'll be reporting back to her how your leg's doing, and she'll be in to see you herself next week."

"Ah weel, that'll hae tae dee," he sighed.

Sometimes confused elderly folk tidied the nurse's equipment away in strange places.

"Where does your nurse keep the dressings packs she brings in for your ulcer dressing, Mrs Stuart?" I asked.

"Fittna' dressings, nursie?" the old lady replied. "I canna tell ye at a'."

After a search I would find a box with dressings, bandages and scissors behind the bread bin in the kitchen cupboard.

During my practical experience I was sometimes allocated a Health Board Mini. There wasn't always a car available and I had to go by bus. I usually ended up walking because I had run out of change to pay the fare.

"Where's the nurse?" a patient would ask. "She should have been here by this time. I've had the water heating all morning for my bath."

In spite of minor hiccoughs like that, I revelled in my new life. Aberdeen is called the Silver City; and when sun shines it certainly lives up to its name. The granite glistens in the northern sunlight. In

May the spires of the horse chestnuts lining the road are beautiful, rhododendron flowers, cherry and almond blossom brighten grey buildings. You turn a corner and look over to the sea, sometimes blue, often steely grey. Standing at a patient's door, I would admire the garden, or listen to a robin's whistle or a blackbird's song.

Aberdeen wins prizes for its flowers in parks and private gardens. Some of the families we visited had beautiful gardens; the men in particular were proud of their handiwork. They often gave me cuttings of their fuschias, but sadly mine never seemed to come on as well.

My elderly patients suffered from diabetes, arthritis, strokes and heart disease, multiple sclerosis and Parkinson's Disease, cancer and leg ulcers. I began to realise how difficult leg ulcers are to cure, and how lonely patients can manipulate the situation because they enjoy the nurse's visits and so don't want the leg to heal.

"That bandage is ower ticht, can you nae just slacken it a bittie?" they would complain, although I explained that support bandaging was the only way to treat them.

"Mr Jack's leg ulcer seems worse this week," I confessed to Liz. "I'm sure he thinks it's because it's me that's doing his dressing and not you."

"These leg ulcers are a total pest," Liz replied. " It's funny though, Margaret, but often you get the ulcer healed and the patient dies soon after."

"Well, perhaps it's just as well Mr Jack's leg isn't healing then," I said with a sigh of relief. "I would hate to have his death on my conscience. He'd look down from heaven and say, 'I'm here because that Margaret cam' and did my leg. I kent she was nae eese!'"

"I doubt if he'll be looking down at you," Liz returned. "Looking up is more like it!"

Eye care after cataract or glaucoma surgery was also part of our work.

"I'm glad now I worked in the Eye Department in Glasgow," I said after Liz told me of a new patient coming home from hospital after cataract surgery.

"Nothing you learn in nursing is ever wasted," Liz agreed.

Finding streets and houses sometimes presented a challenge.

"Map reading and car maintenance would be useful subjects to learn in the college," I said, "sociology and psychology, aren't much use when you're lost in a housing scheme on a foggy night, and whichever way up you hold the map, you can't see the direction to take. Another problem is when vandals ink out the street names so especially in the dark, it's impossible to find where you are."

"Imagine what it would be like away out in the country," Liz said. "And working in an isolated area would be much more difficult, especially in the winter with deep snow to struggle through. You'll hear some stories from your friends when you go back to the College!"

Soon we were back to theoretical work in College where we learnt how to write care plans using the latest models of nursing.

"In nursing, care plans are the order of the day," I told Carol during one of our telephone conversations. "You have to devise how to plan and implement nursing care using a patient centred approach."

"Imagine the likes of Sister Dunn if you said you were using a patient centred approach?" I could tell Carol was smiling ruefully at the memory of the sister who had terrorised us in the days of our training.

"She would say the work centred round her orders, not what the patients want," I said. "The model she wanted was the nurse sitting the patient up in a neatly made bed, having cleaned his mouth, scrubbed his face, rubbed his pressure areas, given him a drink, all at top speed."

"Yes, and then that same nurse should be in the sluice cleaning the bed pans, or in the ward tidying the linen cupboard," Carol went on. "She certainly wasn't sitting talking to the patient to find out his ideas of what nursing care would suit him best!"

"You have to ask patients about their sexual needs – it all goes into the care plan to give a holistic approach."

"That would really put the tin lid on things. Exit the nurse out on her ear with the care plan following her," Carol laughed over the phone.

"Or exit Sister feet first on the mortuary trolley."

At last the time came for the written examination and then we all went our separate ways to city and island to face different challenges and rewards in this new sphere of nursing care.

Chapter 12: The A Team

Now a brand new district nursing sister, I was about to begin a different kind of nursing, which would develop and change as community care became a political issue for better or worse.

District nurses wore a top quality Harris tweed coat, or a lighter weight raincoat, and short sleeved dresses. This uniform was the same throughout the British Isles. Sisters wore royal blue, enrolled nurses dark green, and nursing auxiliaries brown. We all wore little pillbox hats, which would blow away and bowl along the road in the north-east gales!

Do you hide behind a uniform? Health visitors had decided some years previously that wearing a uniform was more of a hindrance than a help in professional relationships. As a district nurse, I personally felt proud to wear a national uniform, and was honoured by the respect that a lot of people showed to the profession. Once again I had a black bag to carry. This time there was definitely no baby inside!

I had already been allocated a sister's post in the west end of Aberdeen, attached to a doctors' practice next door to the secondary school my two sons attended.

"That's great, Mum," they said, "You'll be able to give us lifts to school every day."

"Oh no, I won't," I said, "I'll be using a pool car and it's not insured for me to take passengers, you'll have to keep getting the bus."

The doctors' practice was in an imposing Victorian villa. The district nurses' office was in the attic with beautiful views over the city. The other district nursing sister Muriel welcomed me with one of her typically warm smiles.

"Hi, I'm Muriel. It's nice to meet you, Margaret. It's a right pech running up these stairs. Get your breath back and then we'll hae a wee lookie at the map and you'll see the lay-out of your district."

A large street map of Aberdeen covered one of the walls under the sloping ceiling.

"I visit patients in Torry, Kincorth, King Street and Seaton." Muriel went on. "You'll cover the centre of the town out to the west end faur a' the posh folks bide," she added with a grin. "Come on. I'll introduce you to the staff. You'll find the doctors and receptionists are fine and friendly. Then I'll tak' you roond your patients. If you hae a few days with me you'll easily find your feet. I canna tell you how glad I am you've been sent here. We've been so short staffed I wasna finishing work till the back o' six every nicht. "

District nurses were supposed to work 8.30 a.m. until 5 p.m. By unwritten law we all started at 8 a.m. There were diabetic patients needing insulin before breakfast, people to be got ready for day centres, and a caseload of work that could be got through more easily the earlier you started.

The practice staff consisted of three GP partners, four receptionists and one practice nurse. The community nursing team had two full time health visitors, who looked after the young families in the practice; and two nursing sisters, Muriel and myself, also a part-time auxiliary nurse, Gail and an enrolled nurse called Sarah. Sarah was young, efficient and extrovert. She had been brought up in Derbyshire, and was recently married. She'd failed her driving test, but nothing daunted, she went round her patients on a moped, wearing a crash helmet instead of her hat.

Although the practice was in the leafy west end, the patients lived all over the city. We went from large houses, to old tenements, to multi storey flats and nineteen fifties housing schemes. The patients were retired professors, doctors or teachers, farming folk who had moved into the city, fishing folk, railway workers, factory workers and everything in between.

Some patients defined their condition in three categories: "Nae weel, affa nae weel, or nae weel at a'," This last meant there was really no hope!

There were people who would never dream of going to the doctor except in a dire emergency, others thought they should summon him for every ache or pain.

"I'm over eighty, the doctor should visit me every month," they said.

Muriel advised me to call on the over eighty-fives on a regular monthly basis. Mr Alexander an old man of ninety-eight said to me, "It's all right in your eighties, but when you're in your nineties life is more difficult."

He was a fit man, despite his age. He lived with his sister, who was ninety-six. Her white hair was streaked with yellow from the cigarettes she smoked. Mr Alexander was very deaf and I had to kneel down to speak to him as he sat in his chair. Once I stood up and was aware of black things floating before my eyes. I thought, that's strange, I don't feel dizzy; then I realised they were flies. The house was filthy. Miss Alexander was far too independent to accept my offer of a home help. One day she greeted me with a big sigh.

"What's wrong, Miss Alexander?" I asked.

"I hate housework," she replied with a woebegone expression. "But don't you come here with all this talk about a home help," she added fiercely. "I'm not having anyone from Social Services in my house."

Patients like the Alexanders, even at their advanced age, were the 'well elderly'. Our other patients required varying degrees of nursing care. Their ages ranged from nine to ninety, and the care included all the family.

After our visits we returned to the office to catch up with paperwork and consult with the doctors about patients they had been called out to see on their morning rounds, and patients who had been discharged home from hospital.

"There's a heap of new patients come in," I said. "It's going to be a really busy afternoon. You'll need to give me a shot of your moped, Sarah. You nip through the traffic in a cloud of blue smoke. I used to see you zooming along the road before I started here, " I recalled. "'There goes a district nurse,' I said to myself."

"Yes, a moped's great for getting round the town in a hurry," agreed Sarah. "I hate keeping the patients waiting. I can just hear them saying 'Where's the nurse, I'm needing to get my leg dressed and she's not here yet'. But I'll be in a pool car on Monday," she added.

"So you've passed your test at last!" Muriel and I exclaimed together.

"Yes, I'm so pleased. The old folks will be disappointed, though. They tell their families about the nurse with the crash helmet and they love waving me off on my bike."

So Sarah started driving around in a Mini and we made time for a cup of coffee in the office to celebrate. Gail the auxiliary nurse joined us. She looked at Sarah with a twinkle in her eye.

"I've just come from Union Grove. I was bathing Mrs Smith..."

"Oh no!" Sarah started to laugh. "Did she tell you about last week?"

"You went to the wrong door!"

Speedy Sarah would run into a house, call to the patient, "Good morning, how are you today?" Then to save time she would rush straight into the bathroom to start running the bath water before going into the living room to help the patient through for her bath.

"Yes, I pressed the service button to get in from the street, raced up those old tenement stairs to the second floor landing but I opened the door on the right instead of the one on the left."

"You never did! And then of course you rushed straight into the bathroom as usual..." Gail prompted, while Muriel and I creased up with laughter.

"Yes," said Sarah. "I started running the bath, then I looked about. 'That's funny, those tiles were green last week, they can't just have changed to blue.' Then it dawned on me. I was in the wrong house!"

"So what did you do then?" I asked. "Did the wifie not call the police because there was a burglar trying to drown her in her bath?"

"Well, I pulled the plug out and went into the living room. 'I'm sorry but I'm the nurse for the lady next door. I came to you by mistake,' I said. 'That's a' richt dearie, I ken fine fa you are. Mrs Smith aye tells me aboot her nursie,' the lady said.

"Aye, they a' ken oor cheery wee Sarah," Muriel said.

"Mrs Smith told me we'll have to add her neighbour to our bathing list," Gail said.

Bathing could be hazardous for us nurses. Muriel visited a lady in the early stages of dementia who was very aggressive. Convinced she would be murdered in her bed, she slept with a kitchen knife under her pillow.

Muriel asked, "Would you like to have a bath today?"

The lady replied, "No, but you would," and pushed Muriel in!

"It's just as weel I hadna run the water in already. I thought I'd wait until she'd started to undress herself," Muriel said when she told us the story.

"If you'd been Sarah, the bath would have been full, and you'd have got soaked," I laughed.

Sarah and I visited two old sisters, Daisy and Maggie. They lived alone at home. Daisy could walk with assistance from her bed to her chair, but Maggie had to be lifted bodily. Maggie was totally helpless and confused, Daisy was merely forgetful.

"It's taking longer and longer to get those two washed and dressed in the morning, isn't it Sarah?" I said. "And by the time we do physiotherapy on Maggie's legs to stop her muscles from getting contracted, the day's nearly done."

One Saturday I visited them as usual, and was just driving home at lunchtime – I happened to live in their street – when I noticed that there was an ambulance outside the old ladies' door.

"That's strange, they were fine when I left," I thought. "I'd better see what's going on."

I went inside the house to find a doctor and two ambulance men trying to discover which of them needed care more than the other. Daisy had phoned for help because she'd forgotten they'd been got up and been washed and fed in the morning.

"I phoned the doctor because you've been such a time coming. 'Where's that nurse?' I said to Maggie. It's not good enough leaving us here alone," Daisy said to me in an aggrieved voice.

"But Daisy, I was here for nearly an hour this morning, getting you both up. Look, you're both dressed and there's the tray of food your home help put out for your lunch," I replied. "You shouldn't have called out an ambulance you know. You surely don't want to go to hospital."

"Oh, no, Maggie and I want to stay here at home, don't we Maggie?" Daisy said. "I'm sorry to have bothered you all. I'm a bit forgetful at times." Daisy looked shamefaced.

"Dinna worry, my quine," one of the ambulance men reassured her. "So long as ye're baith a' richt, there's nae hairm deen. We'll be awa' noo."

"I'll be back later in the afternoon, Daisy," I said. "And don't worry, I shan't forget about you. You'll keep her right, won't you Maggie?" I smiled at Maggie, knowing she didn't have a clue what was happening.

"It's so nice to have all these visitors dearie," Maggie said. "It cheers us up to have company. You sit down and I'll go into the kitchen to make us all our fly cuppie o' tea."

Daisy used to phone the only answering machine the community nurses had. It was in a clinic and the patients were given the number to use in an emergency.

"Why won't you speak to me?" she would demand, "Where's the nurse? My sister needs to go to bed." She could never understand why the machine wouldn't reply.

Daisy wasn't the only one to get mixed up with the modern technology. Once I heard a distraught voice on the answer machine, "Help, help I need a nurse." Another call I remember was, "Mary, it's that damt machine. Faur's ma glesses, Mary? Hurry up and bring them tae me" And that was all.

But with no name or telephone number there was nothing I could do about either call.

Eventually Daisy and Maggie both needed two nurses three times a day, and home helps twice a day, as Daisy too became frailer.

I felt very concerned about them and told their GP about it at a team meeting.

"Alan, those two old sisters are taking up hours of nursing time. They're in need of twenty-four-hour care now."

"Yes, I think we've reached the end of the road with the amount of care we can offer," Alan agreed. "But Daisy won't readily agree to go into hospital, and she's still able to sign a consent form herself. I'm afraid we'll have to wait until something occurs to warrant their admission."

Daisy developed severe back pain as she had osteoporosis and Alan arranged for them to be admitted to a geriatric ward.

"I feel guilty every time I pass their door," I said to Sarah. "I feel we've let them down. Come on and visit them in hospital with me."

"OK," she agreed. "I wonder if they'll know us."

In fact they were quite happy in the hospital lying in beds next to each other just as they had done at home.

"I'm glad we went, Sarah," I said, "I can pass their house with an easier mind."

Twenty years later, I still look out for the snowdrops Daisy had planted in her front garden, and as their delicate flowers appear in the snow, I remember the two old sisters with an affectionate smile as I walk past their door.

We visited other old confused folk who needed help with medication. Some of them could still go out and about. Teenie told Muriel all about the new supermarket that had just opened.

"That's a really fine placie," she said. "They gie you a ticket and shout your number like at the bingo. And the next you ken, you've won a quarter o' biled ham to tak hame."

Once Muriel got tickets for a concert of Scottish songs.

"Come on, let's all of us tak some o' oor aul craters to the Music Hall. It'll gie them a night oot and help remind them of the aul days. Teenie will ken a' the songs."

We invited some of the less frail patients and drove them to the show in our cars. Some of them discovered they were long lost friends.

"Div ye min' we baith worked wi' the fish?" Betty asked Aggie.

"Aye, fairly that. It was the time o' the war." Aggie replied. "I min' I eesed to tak' a fine haddock hame to my mither. I hid it in my knickers."

"They were the guid days," the two old ladies both agreed. "And it's thanks tae oor nursie Muriel we've met up again."

"Aye, my man and I ca' her the bonny lass o' Fyvie," Aggie said.

Even in the dim light of the concert hall we all had a laugh at Muriel's blushes. The next day Muriel said to Teenie, who had enjoyed every minute of her evening out,

"That was a fine night last night." But of course Teenie had forgotten all about it.

"Did you hae a nicht oot wi' your man?" Teenie replied. "I was in my bed at the back o' nine, there was naething fine at a' on the T.V. I dinna ken hoo they get awa' wi' makking us aul' pensioners pay sae muckle for wir licence."

Sarah became pregnant, and left us to have her family. She was a breath of fresh air in the lives of the elderly, frail people she visited, and nothing was too much trouble for her. After she left us, I took over most of her work and discovered then how much extra help she had given.

"'Where's that young nurse? You're bringing in my prescription right enough, but she aye went tae the chemist for my peels, and I'm needing a pint of milk from the shoppie next door an' a'," they said.

After she'd had her baby, Sarah went back to work part time in the evening, settling people down for the night. She once put the wrong person to bed. There is a little old fishing village in Aberdeen with a North Square and a South Square. Sarah went to the wrong address and valiantly tried to persuade the woman who lived there – who happened to be an alcoholic – that she really ought to go to bed. Meantime the correct client was phoning the night sister complaining her nurse was late in coming to put her to bed!

"Where's the nurse? She should have been to me an hour ago. This service just isn't good enough," an irate voice spoke on the night sister's answer phone.

We heard the story from our new colleague, twenty-four-year-old Sheila whom I had met on the District Nursing Course. By coincidence, Sheila's aunt had been the night sister who had taken the phone call that evening.

"That's the way I ken aboot Sarah, " Sheila explained. "How are things, Margaret? It's right fine to see you again."

"It's fine to see you too, Sheila. We never thought when we were on the course we'd work together on the district. We're a great team, here."

"We call ourselves the A. Team, " Gail put in, " I suppose everyone thinks they have the best team of nurses. But we really are the best!

"I'm glad I've been sent here then," Sheila said. "When we finished the course, I started to work out in Dyce. Then last week, my nurse manager moved me here. 'Last in, first out' she said."

"It's really fine to hae you here," Muriel assured her. "We were short staffed again wi' Sarah leaving."

A few weeks after Sheila joined us a new auxiliary nurse called Evelyn was added to our team. We five nurses, Muriel, Sheila, Gail. Evelyn and I stayed together working for the same practice for the next ten years. Evelyn was a Gaelic speaker who brought West Coast exuberance to the understated North East. She had trained as a nurse in Glasgow in the fifties, but had to leave before finishing her training in order to nurse her invalid mother. She had then married, had four children and worked in hospital and in the community in various parts of Scotland.

She always signed her name "OBE."

"Why do you write OBE?" Gail asked her. "The patients all think you've been awarded a real OBE. "

"You tell them it stands for Our Boss Evelyn, and then they'll understand, " Evelyn smiled mysteriously.

"Hey, Evelyn, you and I know what else it stands for – oil, bath and enema," I said, laughing. "After four babies you know all about that."

"I sure do, and that's when I started it, when I was working in a maternity hospital, and it just seems to have stuck."

We soon learnt that Evelyn had rather quaint phrases she used in conversation, and that she never could remember the names of the folk she'd visited or where they lived. When she was filling up her records she'd say, "I was at Mrs Boom Boom in such and such street".

One day she called on a lady named Mrs Fraser who had fallen and dislocated her shoulder. Evelyn helped her wash and dress. She reached for a skirt.

"Is this the one you're wearing today?" Evelyn asked pleasantly.

"Yes," came the reply. "It's an old one. I've had it for ages. I bought it at F and M's."

This was the abbreviation for Fraser and Miller's, a long established family run department store.

"I used to like that store," said Evelyn. "But it's really gone downhill lately."

To her amazement, Mrs Fraser glared at her fiercely. "Is that your opinion of the best department store in Aberdeen? Actually I own it."

"Didn't you realise who the patient was?" I asked when Evelyn told me later.

"In the name of the wee man, Margaret, you know what I'm like with names. I thought it was Mrs Duthie in Fraser Avenue, not Mrs Fraser in Duthie Place," she said.

"Och well, that's you off the list for the free pairs of tights from F and M's," I said. "Never mind, I'll share mine with you."

But Mrs Fraser must have been too offended to come up with any free gifts, because once her arm was better that was the last we heard of her!

A while later it was my turn not to recognise a famous Aberdonian. Mr Scott had become bedridden with a bad back. He lived in one of the most elegant of all Aberdeen districts. I got out of my car and walked up a long drive, carrying a commode and plastic urinal. Mrs Scott ushered me into a beautiful oak panelled hall, and up a sumptuously carpeted stair. I followed her still carrying my incongruous load.

"Good afternoon Mr Scott," I said to the rather frail elderly man lying in bed. "I'm the district nurse from the surgery. How can I help you?"

"I don't think you can do anything," he replied. "I'm waiting for the physiotherapist to come from Pittodrie, and I'm sure he'll sort me out."

"Oh, in that case I'll leave you these things and come back tomorrow morning to see how you are." I said goodbye and went out to my car. Back in the office I said to Muriel,

"Alan asked me to do a home assessment today. The patient, Mr Scott lives in a lovely house, one of the nicest I've ever been to. When I got there Mr Scott said he didn't need me. He was waiting for the physio from Pittodrie. Why on earth do you think he'd be wanting Aberdeen football club's physio?"

"Did you nae ken fa that was?" Muriel laughed. "He's the owner of the Aberdeen football club. He'll maybe sign a photo of the Dons for your loons."

"Jings and crivvens, I'm not the only numpty who can't put a name to a face!" Evelyn said with great satisfaction.

Evelyn's humour and professional manner kept her on top of most situations, but one time she almost let herself down by giving out a yell of astonishment – almost but not quite. She went into a house, knowing that the lady, Mrs Watt, had died the previous afternoon, sitting peacefully in her armchair while her daughter was out shopping. Miss Watt was totally distraught at her mother's death. When the undertakers came with the coffin she had refused to let them put the old lady's body into it.

"That coffin's not good enough for my mother, you'll have to get a better one," she demanded.

So when Evelyn went into the living room, there, suspended in a state of apparent levitation was the body of old Mrs Watt, draped in a sheet and lying on a trestle, looking as though she were ascending up to heaven.

"Great Gordon Highlanders! I got such a fright, my blood ran cold," Evelyn told us. "I thought it was a ghost I was seeing. I tell you, I was nearly needing a coffin too!"

"You must have got a real fright" I sympathised. "Here, have a cup of coffee, strong and black to restore your nerves."

"Thanks, Margaret. I think I will. I'll never forget seeing the old mother flying up to heaven in that white sheet as long as I live," Evelyn declared. "Auchtermuchty, Dobbie's Loan and Govan by the Sea, she'll haunt me for the rest of my days!"

So we had our OBE to keep us going, and if laughter is the best medicine, Evelyn certainly administered it in generous doses – to us as well as to her patients.

Chapter 13: Houses - and the people inside them

A row of houses looks so different once you're on the inside. A grey granite Victorian terraced house keeps its secrets firmly hidden behind its solid front door. Inside it can be smart and fashionable, or old and dilapidated. One house I visited was definitely not in the top league for modernity. Every room still had bells to ring for the servants, but where were they a hundred years on? The house had once been heated throughout by coal fires, in the past all the rooms would have been warm and cosy, but now it was freezing cold with one electric fire in the living room. Two elderly sisters, retired teachers, lived there. It had been their father's house; their family had been the sole occupants since it was built in the eighteen nineties.

The elder Miss Robertson came on our list.

"Margaret, I've got a real problem lady for you to sort out," Alan told me in the surgery one day. "Her name is Miss Robertson. She suffers from osteoarthritis and is extremely immobile. She lives with her elderly sister who can't help her at all and between you and me the pair of them fight like cat and dog. Our Miss Robertson has been in hospital to try to get her walking again. Before that she was stuck in her upstairs bedroom unable to go to the toilet, even though it's just across the landing."

"However did she manage?" I wondered.

Alan looked slightly embarrassed. "It was ghastly, Margaret! The environmental health people had to clean the place up. Now she's coming home, Miss Robertson has reluctantly agreed to sleep downstairs – the hospital staff explained there's no way her sister could care for her unless she does."

"If there's no love lost between them it's not likely there'll be any TLC in this house," I commented. "However, one thing we can do on a practical level is to bring in a commode."

"Her sister has already asked for one to be delivered before Miss Robertson is discharged," Alan went on. "I'd be glad if you could use all your charms to rehabilitate this lady, and organise her nursing care."

"Not that old witch!" Pat, one of our receptionists at the practice said to me when she heard Alan's story, "How I hated her at school! I had her for French and German. She was a real bully. I don't envy you, Margaret. If she hasn't mellowed with age you'll never get her to listen to a word you say."

Miss Robertson was indeed a formidable character who refused to change her ways.

"This is the drawing room I'm residing in, not the bedroom: all the bedrooms in my home are upstairs," she said in her best schoolteacher's voice.

In this once elegant drawing room, Miss Robertson now slept on an ancient bed settee with an antiquated horsehair mattress. Her commode stood beside the settee and we battled to get her on to it.

"A person with osteoarthritis should be allowed to stay in her bed!" she complained.

"Miss Robertson's quite a handful isn't she? How's the rehabilitation going, Margaret?" Alan asked.

"Alan, she's really difficult," I sighed. " All she wants to do is stay in that saggy, baggy old bed. She scratches and hits whenever I try to help her up. I've decided to ask Evelyn and Gail to do the visits with me. There's safety in numbers!"

"That's a good idea," Alan approved. "I've thought about prescribing tranquillisers but that will increase her risk of falling. I would like you to do some blood tests. We'll check her haemoglobin and her vitamin B12 levels to see if she's anaemic."

"Would you like me to check her thyroid levels too, Alan? It could be something like a low thyroid that's causing her aggression." I suggested.

"We'll do a thorough examination, then. You go and look out the biggest needle and syringe you can find – that'll show her who's boss," Alan joked.

Miss Robertson's blood tests were all normal.

"It's her nature, not any illness that makes her so bad. I still shudder when I think of her, she put me off French and German for life," Pat the receptionist said when the blood reports came back.

"Help my kilt, that old lady Robertson's a problem," Evelyn agreed. "You know she hasn't got any decent clothes?"

"I think the environmental folk had to chuck away most of her things when they blitzed the place out," I said, "I bought some clothes at a sale of work and took them in. She nearly ate me. 'I don't want any of those rags. How dare you imply I need charity.' I hid them amongst her old tatty things, and her home help, Jessie puts them out one at a time for her."

"I brought in a mohair stole," Evelyn added. "It's freezing cold in that house. The next day she was all huddled in that ancient fox fur coat, and the stole was bundled down the back of the chair. Sometimes you get fed up trying to be nice to folk."

"You're not kidding. That fur coat dates from the nineteen thirties. I think it can walk over to the bed settee by itself. Never mind, Evelyn, she's a lot mellower since you and Gail started going together to her. She thinks she's special having two nurses to attend to her; your company cheers her up."

Gail and Evelyn did their best to brighten her life.

"We're having a birthday party for Miss Robertson tomorrow afternoon," Gail told me. "Would you like to come too? We've asked Jessie and the neighbour down the road."

"You're so good to her, both of you. And you're both doing this on your afternoon off," I said.

"Ach, well, we'll get our reward in heaven," Evelyn laughed. "Though I don't know if Miss R. will be there to see it."

It was great to see Miss Robertson with an elaborate party hat Gail had made, sipping sherry with the lady next door, and getting all giggly!

Miss Robertson stayed in her own home for several months longer with daily visits from nurses and home helps. In the end, she had to be admitted to hospital.

We nurses weren't sorry to take her off our books. Such a beautiful house on the outside, we agreed; lovely chairs covered with tapestries she'd embroidered herself, and the elegant staircase covered with a royal blue carpet of her own making, but what a nightmare to try to care for such a difficult person!

Another Victorian home in the genteel west end was owned by Mrs Bates, a widow who lived with her son Richard. He suffered from schizophrenia. Mrs Bates had been a theatre sister, but bladder problems, on top of years of coping with her son's intractable illness had got her down and she had totally given up. The gracious large rooms were dilapidated and freezing cold. Mrs Bates used to lock herself into her bedroom to be away from her son.

"What a shame for Mrs Bates to cower away in her bedroom like that," I said to Alan. "Can Richard not get respite care? A spell in hospital might improve his condition."

"He comes up to the surgery regularly for his anti-psychotic injections, and he's relatively stable at the moment," Alan replied. "Schizophrenia is such a devastating illness, Margaret, families become so isolated."

"His mother's incontinence makes her withdraw as well. She doesn't want to admit she's got a problem. I would like her to try without a catheter because she has continual urinary infections. I'm encouraging her to drink cranberry juice. I read a scientific paper saying that it alters the acidity of the urine, enabling the bacteria to be flushed away."

"When I was a theatre sister in Saint Bartholomew's hospital, I never thought I would need a district nurse," Mrs Bates said on my next visit. "I can't go without a catheter, though."

"Would you not try to monitor your bladder control yourself Mrs Bates?" I asked. "Long term catheterisation isn't the only answer. I could give you charts to fill in and we could refer you to the continence advisor. "

"No, no, I can't change my routine. When I was a theatre sister the surgeons used to ask my advice. I'm not going to listen to any continence woman. I don't even have a home help. Richard won't let strangers into the house," Mrs Bates became quite agitated.

I remembered how Liz, my practical work teacher told me that in the patient's home the nurse is the guest. Although I could suggest ways to help this lady there was no guarantee she would follow my advice.

"Tell me about Richard, Mrs Bates," I changed the subject. "Has he been ill for long?"

"My son became ill when he went away to Australia with the navy. It had always been his ambition to go to sea, but then he broke down. It's been twenty years you know, such a waste of a young man's life."

"It's not easy for you," I sympathised.

"Richard was such a clever boy when he was young. His father died just before he joined the navy. Perhaps that had something to do with his illness. You know, Nurse, the treatment for schizophrenia is still in the dark ages, and there's such a stigma attached to it."

Mrs Bates died suddenly in her sleep some months after our conversation. After she died Richard was given a supported flat, but he couldn't cope alone and was admitted to the psychiatric hospital. He committed suicide whilst he was an in-patient, a tragic end to a sad life.

Some of the homes our patients lived in were beautifully kept with lovely furniture and every latest gadget. But some were very different! Ivy, who had spent years as a prostitute round the docks, had a one-bedroom flat in a 1930s' housing scheme.

"I was at Ivy at the weekend," I said to Muriel. "What a poor wifie and such a filthy home."

"I ken, Margaret. It's a shame to see an aul body living like that."

The only clean thing was the bed. This typical hospital bed with its high metal frame and back rest had come from the nurses' equipment store, as had the starched white bed linen. Even in the1980s, washing machines or hot water in the home were not to be taken for granted.

The hospital linen service delivered clean sheets to the patients' homes each week

"Young loons on community service for criminal offences were supposed to redecorate the house," Muriel told me. "The walls were black with grease, you wouldna' ken there was flooery wallpaper underneath. They managed to strip the walls but they couldna' stand Jock. A' that swearing! Ivy swears back at him but naebody can mak oot a word she says. That's why folk ca' her 'Snuffy Ivy!'"

"Yesterday I left the house with my ears ringing from their foul language. I took a great gulp of fresh air and just across the road there were all the folk going into church in their Sunday best. What a different world from one side of the road to the other even in that little housing scheme," I commented.

"Torry folk still mind on 'Snuffy' Ivy, she aye wore a blonde wig and lime green trousers," Muriel reminisced.

"I used to see her with that wig and those trousers when I was waiting for the bus home from the Castlegate," I remembered. "She won't be there again, that's for sure. It's all she can do to walk from her bed to her chair."

A month later, on my next weekend on duty I learned that Ivy had been found dead in her bed with Jock lying beside her corpse, quite oblivious to the fact she was stone cold.

Once you have nursed patients inside the different houses in a town you can never walk by without thinking of them. Mrs Walker, well in her seventies, lived in a tenement flat with no hot water, no bath and an outside toilet. I used an old tin basin to give her a wash. She slept in the kitchen in an old-fashioned box bed. Her handicapped son, Jimmy, in his fifties lived with her.

"Old Mrs Walker's such a poor soul," I said to Muriel and Sheila when we were in the office in the afternoon doing our paperwork. "There's no comfort in that home. Jimmy does his best and always has a kettle of water boiling, but he can barely look after himself."

"I ken, " Sheila said. "I'm nae happy wi' that strange chiel. I am aye wondering faur his hands will go next when I'm bending over that low bed."

"I know, you need eyes in the back of your head with him," I agreed. " I try to help him sort out his medication. He's on a heap of pills, and there's bottles lying everywhere. I've brought in some egg boxes so we can put each day's pills in the different sections. But I hate thinking of Mrs Walker in that poor place She won't have a home help. She says Jimmy can manage all the housework."

"It's affa' tae think folk are still living wi' nae hot water and an ootside loo. It's like auld Bella, the wifie I go to up in Rosemount. But if folk winna let the council modernise their hooses, there's nae much we can do," Muriel joined in.

Mrs Walker was diagnosed with tuberculosis. She was admitted to hospital and made a good recovery, but insisted on going back home to the same conditions. Today the tenements in her street are all modernised with inside toilets and showers. I see them advertised as "a desirable flat suitable for the first time buyer".

Muriel's patient, Bella lived in a tenement flat with an old range that no longer worked. Her home help heated up her dinner on an electric ring. There was a cold water tap in the kitchen, where Bella slept in a box bed. Her toilet was outside, so she used a commode. Even in the middle of June Bella wore seven cardigans to keep herself warm. It was a time consuming exercise undressing her to give her a wash!

Bella had a leg ulcer. Muriel encouraged her to sit with her feet up to try to improve her circulation, but Bella continued to pull her chair right in front of her electric fire, scorching her legs in her effort to keep warm.

"Bella's got tartan legs," Muriel informed us. "It's nae easy to use an aseptic technique when I'm dressing her leg ulcer. I bring in antiseptic wipes for my hands."

"There's nowhere to lay oot the dressings packs and sterile scissors," Sheila agreed. "The last wee student nurse I had wi' me couldna believe it. 'Where's the dressings pack to go?' she asked. 'We hae to improvise' I told her. 'Newspaper laid oot ower an aul chair works just as weel.' She was shocked, but I explained that Bella probably has less infection than if she was in the hospital."

Bella singed her hair going to bed by candlelight. Evelyn who came in to wash her, bought her a cheap bedside light from the Oxfam shop so that she wouldn't need to use candles after switching off her main light switch at the door. She wouldn't use it. "That's too grand for me," she'd said.

Evelyn and Muriel both tried to persuade Bella to move to sheltered housing.

"You'll hae to ging soon," Muriel said "Your hoose is on the list to be knockit doon"

"Dinna worry, I'm the second phase, the mannie fae the cooncil showed me the plans," Bella replied.

But at long last Bella was moved. In her new sheltered flat she always walked about with a net bag stuffed full of newspaper attached to her zimmer frame.

"I'm still worried aboot Bella," said Muriel. "She canna work her security system, so she aye leaves her door unlocked. I tell her it's nae safe, she could be burgled. I've shown her what way it works but she's so thrawn, she winna listen."

"It's the same with those old newspapers. What a weight to humph about on her zimmer!" Evelyn added. " I told her I was going to put them out to the bucket. You should have seen her face! I can't think why she's so attached to them."

One day the mystery of the newspapers was explained. Muriel's fears were realised and Bella *was* burgled.

"A man called on Bella pretending he was frae the cooncil; he'd come to check her heating. He saw her purse lying on her kitchen table and went off wi' it," Muriel told us.

The police were called. They told Bella they would need to do a thorough search of her things to check if anything else had been taken. To everyone's amazement they discovered that she had several thousand pounds hidden among the newspapers in her net bag. All these years she'd been living so frugally and never spending her pension. She hadn't allowed her home help to put her money in the bank or post office.

"Bella had that muckle money that she shouldna hae been getting her home help for free," Muriel continued her story. "It's a shame she didna spend it on herself instead of living a' those years with nae comforts in that caul aul hoose."

So, Victorian villas and tenements, modern sheltered accommodation, 1950s' housing schemes, high rise blocks: we visited them all!

Lizzie lived in a real period piece of 1930s' architecture. Lizzie was nearly a hundred years old and was full of stories of her girlhood.

"I was twelve years aul when I left the school to go and work for a fermer nearby," Lizzie told me. "During the First World War a' the men left to fight in France. I chaved awa' at their work in the fields as weel as daeing a' the work in the hoose."

"You can see by your hands you've worked hard all your days, Lizzie," I replied.

"But ye ken it wasna a' hard work, we made oor ain entertainment. I min' on twa brithers fa bed in a wee hoosie doon the road. They werena' the full shilling so they couldna ging awa tae the War. They were grand singers and aye sang as they traivelled aboot the place. The song they sang maist was the Bonny Banks o' Loch Lomond, so a'body ca'd ane o' them Bonny and the ither ane Banks. Aye me, life's nae the same noo richt enough!"

"No, nobody leaves school at twelve to go out to work," I commented.

"Aye, but Mr Michie the fermer was guid tae me. When he selt the ferm and cam to Aiberdeen tae bide I went wi' him and his sister as their housekeeper."

"Why did he decide to come into town rather than stay in the country?" I wondered.

Her answer was brief and to the point. "Inside sanitation."

After the farmer and his sister died, Lizzie's younger brother Eddie moved in to live with her. He was a mere youth of eighty-five! Lizzie was related to the composer Edward Grieg and often had enquiries from Norwegian people about her forbears.

"I canna keep up wi' a' the folk speiring aboot my folks noo," she said. "I'd lo'e to help but I'm ower aul'. I tell them tae ging tae the cemetery at Rathen, that's faur they'll find a' the names on the tombs. It's through my mither's side there's the connection but I'm nae able to spik tae veesitors noo, I'm sae hard o' hearing."

She'd learned to drive in the 1930s and was proud she'd passed her driving test.

"You didna need to pass your test in those days, but I thocht it would be best to tak it and mak sure I was daeing a'thing richt. I stoppit driving when I was ninety, but I fairly missed my car, it wis an Armstrong Sidley," Lizzie told me proudly.

Just after reaching her hundredth birthday Lizzie fell and broke both her arms. I went up to the hospital to visit her and came away feeling so sad that this great old lady should finish her days in such a way. A way of life bound up by times and seasons, hard work and contentment died with her.

One house we visited in a 1950s' scheme was in pristine condition. The bathroom was modern, the décor was the latest fashion and the furniture was immaculate. The family in this lovely house coped gallantly with severe health problems.

Old Mrs Mitchell had osteoarthritis. She lived with her daughter, Mary and Mary's two grown up sons. Evelyn and I both visited to care for Mrs Mitchell. We also gave support to the family.

"Mrs Mitchell is a gem," Evelyn said. "She's in a lot of pain but she's always so cheery."

"They're such fine folk," I agreed. "Her daughter Mary never complains either, although she has her hands full with her mother to care for and both those sons as well."

The oldest son, Tommy, now in his twenties had suffered from rheumatoid arthritis since the age of six. He was a pale thin lad who often lay in bed all day.

"Tommy gets a bit depressed at times. He would dearly like to work but he's nae able," Mary told me.

"Your younger lad, Billy never seems depressed," I observed. "He's always so cheery, and so are you, Mary."

"Well, I have to keep going. It's nae easy sometimes, especially when Billy's having a bad time with fits."

Billy had accidentally been shot in the head when he was twenty-one. He was left with some of the bullet in his brain and was paralysed down his right side. His speech was poor and he had developed severe epilepsy.

"Billy used to work in a shop that sold shot guns and fishing tackle," Mary told Evelyn and me.

"One of his friends came in, picked up a gun and pressed the trigger, never realising the gun was loaded. Billy was right in the line of fire. The thing that makes me bitter is that lad never came to see Billy afterwards or ask how he was."

"He probably couldn't face what he'd done," I replied. "But you've been left to cope, and you know, Mary, you're all so welcoming and your home's so beautiful. It's a pleasure for us to come here."

"Especially for your coffee," Evelyn added. "And to visit your loo! I'm putting you in for the Loo of the Year award!"

A few weeks later old Mrs Mitchell had some good news.

"We've been invited to a wedding in Zimbabwe," she told me excitedly. "We're all going. I'll be helped at the airport by the staff there. Billy's been looking up the flights on Ceefax. He's in his element."

"That's great," I replied. "That lovely climate will help Tommy and you with your arthritis."

"I'm going on safari," Billy said.

"Put me in your rucksack!" I laughed. "I'm coming too!"

"They'll be away for six weeks," I told Evelyn later.

"Oh, michty me," she said in mock horror. "Their loo is one of the ones that I've got marked out to visit in an emergency. I'll have to cross my legs now for six weeks!"

When they returned from their holiday, Tommy was so much better he was able to get a job; his morale improved as well as his health. Evelyn got her comfort stop back and we were all happy!

Chapter 14: "But there's nae bonny laddie will tak me awa'..."

Some old men still bore injuries sustained in the First World War. "Isn't it dreadful, these old men have been disabled for most of their lives because they were wounded in the 1914-18 war," I remarked one day. My mind went back to the old man who had come up to the Casualty in Glasgow to have his wound dressed for so many years.

Many of these elderly gentlemen were simply glad they'd survived. Mr Gibson had lost his right arm at the battle of the Somme at the age of 18. Now at 86 he still considered he was fortunate because having been invalided out of the army he had escaped more of the horrors of the trenches.

Mr Gibson had Parkinson's Disease but it was his wife who was having health problems. She was becoming confused and kept falling. Her one-armed husband was unable to lift her and so they used to phone for the police to come and pick her up whenever she fell.

"I do enjoy the police coming to help me, they're such handsome young men," Mrs Gibson told me one morning, after she'd called them out in the middle of the night.

"I'm sure they'd be delighted to hear you say that," I said with a smile. "Most of their customers aren't so pleased to see the police at the door."

Another long-term casualty was Mr Thomson who had his jaw blown off in the same war. He'd been patched up somehow and spent the next seventy years managing with no teeth or gums. He and his wife had lived in the same ground floor tenement flat all their married life. The printed rules for order and cleanliness in the tenement were displayed at the entrance to the common stair and this old couple obeyed them to the letter.

These rules included no running on the stairs, no children playing and no animals. Mr and Mrs Thomson still scrubbed the stairs and polished the worn linoleum until it gleamed.

"This stair has aye been kept spotless, but the young ones nowadays dinna bother to sweep or clean. We ask them tae tak their turn but they dinna pay a blind bit of notice," Mr Thomson lamented. "Me and the wife are the anes that keep up the cleaning but we're nae so able and it maks us sad to see oor flair in sic a sotter."

"I know Mr Thomson," I commiserated. "You sacrificed so much for your country when you were their age."

"I ken, lassie, I havena had a proper denner since, I canna chew a fine bit o' beef at a'. These young students and their bidey - ins are all vegetarians and wouldna eat an Aberdeen Angus if it sat richt doon in front of them at the table. Oor Rabbie was richt enough wi' his Selkirk Grace," and he quoted, "Some hae meat and canna eat..."

Mr Davidson had won the Military Cross in the First World War, and in the Second he had been in the Home Guard in London during the Blitz. He described going to a dance hall that had been bombed and seeing bits of bodies sticking to remains of glass chandeliers.

"You know, Nurse, I found civilian deaths much harder to cope with than the horrors I witnessed in the trenches. It all seemed so much worse in ordinary homes, very indecent somehow," he looked sad as he spoke.

The old ladies too had experienced what war could do. So many were single – the young men had all perished in the carnage of war. One elderly lady, Alice explained, "The older women took the men when the lads came home from the war, so there were none left for us."

Alice was one of seven sisters; only two of the seven had ever married. Alice lived with three unmarried sisters in a two bed-roomed house; two sisters sleeping together in one room and two in the other. The four of them came on my books when the oldest sister was dying. I continued to visit the other three sisters for many years. Annie was going blind, Gertie had a colostomy, so she too needed support from the nursing service. Alice was the fittest of the three. She had a wry sense of humour and I always left the house with a smile on my face.

"Folk must think I'm daft, walking down the front path grinning to myself," I said to Muriel. "But that Alice is such a character, she's always up to something that gives me a laugh."

"They're a great lot, they'll stick at nothing," Muriel said. "I visited them last week when you were off. I couldna see them in the hoose so I went oot into the gairden. A voice cried doon to me. I lookit up and saw Alice richt up a tree sawing a branch. 'Come awa doon frae there afore you fa', ' I called, and I tried to gie her a hand, but she managed fine hersel'. I hope I'm as fit if I ever live to her age."

The next time I visited the house I found Alice halfway up the chimney.

"I'm busy sweeping the lum," she explained, emerging covered in soot.

On another occasion I was driving along the road and noticed the three of them walking to the shops. Suddenly Alice disappeared amongst the bushes at the entry to an old folk's home. I stopped to see if they were all right.

"I just needed a pee," she said.

"It must be your water pills," I said sympathetically, "They can be a real pest can't they? You've still got quite a walk up the hill. Can I give you a lift home?"

The three of them piled into my car. I think they were glad of the lift though they wouldn't admit it.

"I was planning to visit you anyway to see how you're doing," I said. "How are you getting on with your new colostomy bags, Gertie?"

"I'm nae doing too badly. I had a visit from the stoma nurse yesterday. She's coming to see me again. I said to her not to come next week," Gertie said. "We're going awa' on the bus to Ballater."

"We thought maybe the Queen was needing some company, she must get lonely in that grand castle. We use our pensioners' tickets and it's a fine cheap day out," Alice added.

They all went into a home together when they became too frail to cope independently any more.

* * *

"We've been really busy lately," Sheila said one day in the office. "But things have quietened doon. Let's go out for lunch tomorrow."

"Good idea! There are plenty of fast food places at this end of the town," Gail remarked.

"I can't believe I've been here a year already," Evelyn said over sticky toffee pudding." I really didn't think I would stay, you know. I was so worried about finding my way around. All I knew of Aberdeen was the shops in Union Street."

"Mind your first day, and you went oot wi' me in that aul car I drove then?" Muriel asked her.

"I'll never forget it. I sat down in the passenger seat, you turned a corner and I shot back the full length of the car. I thought my last hour had come," Evelyn remembered.

"I couldna think fit had happened. One minute you were there and the next you'd disappeared, " Muriel said.

"It was worse when I went out with Margaret," Evelyn went on. "She's a low flying aircraft, that one. I had my eyes shut half the time. 'Hold on a cotton picking minute,' I told her. But she's getting better," she added. "I only screamed three times the last time she drove me."

"Well, it's these Minis, they don't like going slow," I said. "My boys say, 'Mum wanted to be a formula one racing driver but her eyesight's not good enough, so she became a district nurse.'"

"Now we're all together, I've got news for you," Sheila said, "I'm going to be married in the summer."

"In the name of the wee man, don't tell me Donnie's got round to popping the question at last!" Evelyn laughed. "I was going to have a word in his ear, he's been so long about it. We'll have a real teuchter wedding when you get hitched."

"But no black cats for good luck," I said. "A big black cat gave me a real fright today. It was Mrs Ford's, you know, the dottled lady we get ready for the day centre every morning."

"Yes, she's so confused she doesn't even recognise her two sons who look after her," Gail replied.

"Her sons thought the cat had gone in next door," I went on with my story. " I opened the drawer in her dressing table to look for her clothes and out sprang the cat. I don't know who got the biggest fright, me or Smoky!"

"I would have jumped out of my skin too," Evelyn put in. "And I'm very fond of Smoky. It's strange isn't it, though she's so confused, Mrs Ford knows all the old songs and hymns off by heart."

"If I want her to stand up I get her to sing 'Stand up, stand up for Jesus'. It always works. She jumps to her feet in a moment," I laughed.

"What's the song she sings about Queen Mary?" Gail asked. "I'd never heard it before."

"Oh, that's a real golden oldie. My mother in law sang it to my boys when they were small. It goes like this:

> *Queen Mary, Queen Mary, my age is sixteen,*
> *My father's a farmer on yonder green,*
> *He's plenty of money to dress me sae braw,*
> *But there's nae bonny laddie tae tak me awa'.*
> *One morning I rose and I looked in the glass,*
> *I said to myself 'what a handsome young lass,'*
> *My hands on my sides and I gave a 'ha, ha',*
> *But there's nae bonny laddie will tak me awa'.*

"That's the one," Gail said. "It reminds me of Alice and her sisters who never got the chance to marry because there were no men left after the First World War."

"Sheila's bonny laddie is ready to tak her awa'," we joked, bringing our thoughts back to the forthcoming wedding.

"Do you think old Granny Leith will be pleased with your news?" Gail asked Sheila. "Though she's so deaf it'll be a job to tell her."

Sheila and Gail visited old Granny Leith twice a day. This lady was a hundred and three years old, very deaf and almost blind. She lived at home with her granddaughter Janet who slept beside the old lady and never had a full night's sleep. Old Granny claimed not to be able to see, but if you came ten minutes later than she expected, she could see the time on the clock all right.

"I'll need a droppie brandy to calm me doon," she would say. "I was lying here thinking 'where's the nurse, she's affa late the day, it's ten minutes to four on the clock'."

Granny Leith was not our only patient to live as long. We had four old ladies whose ages added together totalled four hundred and eight years. Some were more independent than others but nevetheless the families were glad of our support.

"Miss Keith is so dedicated to her old mother and her aunt, who are ninety-six and ninety-eight. She just gets one afternoon off a week with the help of the Crossroads carers you set up for her, Margaret," Evelyn remarked as we walked back to the office after our lunch.

"She looked after her old father too," Gail reminded us. "That was before your time. He was well in his nineties too when he died."

In fact Miss Keith's aunt lived to be ninety-nine and her mother died at the age of one hundred and three; she had devoted all her retirement years to the unselfish care of elderly relatives. Whenever I saw bright holiday postcards on our office notice board I often recalled a conversation I had once had with her.

"It's in the summer I get a bit down," she said. " I haven't had a holiday in years. You nurses tell Mother and me about your holidays; my friends all go away, and all I do is read the post cards. I'm reluctant to put Mother into a home again to give me a break."

"Yes, I remember you got her settled in a home that time you had your operation, but she fell and fractured her femur," I said. "She's done so well to get back on her feet again. It would have been the end of a lot of folk."

Mrs Keith eventually died peacefully at home at the age of one hundred and three, a tribute to the selfless nursing care her daughter had given over so many years. Gail, Evelyn and I felt privileged that we were able to help in her terminal care.

One day we had a phone call from the liaison staff in one of the hospitals. Liaison nurses were responsible for planning the discharge of vulnerable people into the community.

"There's a patient who is desperate to go home. She's really pining, although her husband drives up to see her every single day," the liaison nurse informed me. "She is chair bound with arthritis, she's blind and has a large bedsore which requires twice daily dressings."

"We'll come up and meet her and her husband and discuss what way we can help them," I said. Muriel and I went to the ward to meet the lady and the nurses who were looking after her.

Thus we were introduced to Katie and her husband Andy. For the next six or seven years we would be involved with caring first for Katie and then for Andy as well, two of the most rewarding people I had ever met.

It was agreed that Katie would go home once we got a hospital bed with a special mattress to try to cure the bedsore. Andy was told he could have a home help, but he refused.

"I was a baker to trade," he said. "And I've been keeping the hoose since Katie lost her sight. We'll manage fine."

Andy came from a country area in Strathdon. His mother had died when he was a young boy and his brothers and sisters were separated, some going to Glasgow with one set of grandparents, whilst he went to Aberdeen with the other set.

"My father couldna look efter us because he was a fee'd orra man, and had to move oot to a new ferm at each new term," Andy told me.

Katie's father had died in the First World War, and her widowed mother had very little money.

"I can remember seeing my father before he went away for the last time," Katie told me. "I must only have been three, my brother was just a baby. After that my mother had a hard struggle to bring us up."

Katie's only brother had died young. She and Andy had no family, and she had been in and out of hospital with rheumatoid arthritis since before the days of the NHS.

"You should write a book about hospital life," I used to say to her. "You've seen so many changes over the years."

Because of their lack of family support, we became great friends of this couple. One day Andy was out in the garden hanging out the washing. Evelyn called to him from the back doorstep, "Andy," then when he didn't reply, she went up to him and put her hands across his eyes. "Guess who?" she asked him.

He was so surprised he exclaimed "Jesus Christ!" to which she replied, "No, it's only Evelyn." We often used to laugh about his divine visitation!

Andy refused to have a gardener, although he was becoming increasingly lame with arthritis in his hips.

"Have you never thought about getting some help with your garden, Andy?" I tried to be as tactful as possible, because the garden was looking a bit neglected, but Andy was so independent.

"I did have a lad who came once, but he was nae mair use than a chocolate fireguard. He didna ken the difference between the weeds and the flooers, so I thought 'Na, na Andy, ye'll jist manage awa yersel', and so I have."

Andy and Katie lived right beside Foresterhill hospital, very near to the helicopter landing pad. One day Andy was nearly in tears.

"Come and hae a look at this, Margaret," he said. I followed him out to his garage. "I've been painting a' the ootside of the hoose, and I'd just finished the garage door, when that damt helicopter came. Look at a' the stew that's been blown up on to the wet paint. I'll hae to start a' ower again."

"That's awful," I said, really vexed for him. "What a mess! I'm so sorry, Andy, after all your hard work."

Katie was upset too. "He never stops, he's doing far too much as it is, without starting all that painting again," she said worriedly.

Katie's bedsore took eight months to heal. I dressed it twice a day at first, packing it with the latest alginate dressings, to make sure it healed from within out.

"It's very different from the dressings and lotions we used to use," I said to Evelyn, as she was assisting me one morning. "Remember all those eusol soaks? They're considered far too abrasive to heal wounds nowadays."

"I suppose we have to move with the times," she said, "but some of the old fashioned ways worked as well."

"I'm sure you being here at home with Andy has a lot to do with your wound healing, don't you think Katie?" I added, and we all agreed on that.

Andy and Katie were great Labour supporters. They'd both worked for the Co-op in the 1920s and 30s, and had gone on protest marches in their youth.

Andy had undergone surgery for rectal cancer when he was in his sixties. "They gave me six months to live without the operation, so I thought aboot Katie and went ahead. I've had a colostomy ever since, but that's a sma' price to pay for a' these years o' life," he said.

One day our conversation turned to cigarette smoking.

"I aye likit a fag," Andy said. "But once in the war time I saw Katie standing in a queue. She telt me she'd waited three quarters of an hour for cigarettes. 'That's the last time ye'll hae to do that for me,' I said, and I stoppit smoking there and then."

Finally Andy had a stroke. He was admitted to hospital and died soon after. Katie had to give up her own home and go into long-term care.

"It's sad to think of Katie ending her days blind and lonely, even though she's sitting in a room with other folk, Margaret," Gail told me once after she'd gone in to visit the old lady

"We had some good laughs with her when Andy was alive, but all that's gone now," I agreed. "They didn't have many friends left alive to visit them at home but at least they had each other. It's so often the one who does the caring who goes first."

"The lady in the office at the home said she enjoyed singing some of the old songs recently when they put on a concert, " Gail said to try to be positive.

"Katy used to sing in the Choral Society when they performed the Messiah in the Music Hall before she lost her sight. Music is a good medicine even when someone is feeling sad and isolated," I said.

"Yes," Gail agreed. "Muriel sings bothy ballads to some of the confused folk. It's a great thing to stop them being too agitated. She plays the bagpipes too."

"Even the stone deaf ones would hear them and do a Highland Fling," I laughed.

We cheered ourselves up with the picture of Muriel in her nurse's uniform piping round her district with the patients coming out of their doors, waving their zimmers and marching along behind her.

Chapter 15: Where's the Nurse?

Initially, I used Health Board cars for visits around the city. These Minis were kept locked in the car park behind an imposing granite house, then the main office for the community nurses in Aberdeen, a mile from my home. I cycled up in the morning with my nurse's bag sitting in the basket on the front of my bike.

To collect the car I had to go into the beautiful wood panelled hall and report to an office.

"You have been allocated the car TSA 163V. Here are the keys." So down I went to the car park to find three other cars blocking my Mini. Back upstairs I'd have to go, collect three other sets of keys, manoeuvre three Minis across the car park, go back upstairs with the keys, then down again, give a sigh of relief, get into the car only to find the petrol tank was empty.

"It's a right pain every morning," I complained to Muriel and Evelyn.

"I couldna abide a' that hassle wi' the Crown cars," Muriel said. She and Evelyn used their own cars and claimed mileage.

"I ran out of petrol on Saturday afternoon," I continued. "I'd been working in Torry and Kincorth all morning, and I never noticed I was low in fuel. I was belting back over there in the afternoon, when, oh dear, there I was stuck right in the middle of the Bridge of Dee."

"Trust you, Margaret. You were rushing on too much as usual. You should have waited a cotton picking minute," Evelyn put in. "Only you would get stuck in such a place on a Saturday afternoon. What did you do?"

"A man came and helped to push my car off the bridge. The traffic had built up behind me, so he was glad to get rid of me. Then I phoned David to come with some petrol for me. Luckily he was at home, or I don't know what I'd have done. The time before that I had a student nurse with me when I ran out of fuel. She helped me push my car to the filling station," I continued.

"Help ma Boab, was that the wee girl called Marion?" Evelyn asked. "She looked really tired when I saw her back at the office. No wonder, if she'd been pushing you all over Aberdeen. You'll be reported to the S.P.C.S.N."

"Whatever's that?" Muriel wondered.

"It's the Society for the Prevention of Cruelty to Student Nurses, of course," Evelyn assured us.

"It was only across the road, luckily and we both pushed the car together, " I defended myself. "But I got a nasty surprise when I was bending down to fill up the tank," I added. "A wasp crawled up my skirt and stung me in a very delicate place. I still feel sore when I think of it!"

"Well you got your comeuppance all right then. The good Lord's up in heaven after all," Evelyn replied with a distinct lack of sympathy.

So we all had a laugh at my predicament.

Changes to the system of car use came. We were allowed to take the Health Board Minis home but we couldn't drive them outside working hours, because the insurance didn't cover personal mileage. So I had a car sitting in the street outside my door leaking oil on to the cobbles at the side of the road.

"That Mini needs a proper service. The oil shouldn't be leaking out like that," David said. "It's very dangerous."

"The other day my exhaust fell off as I was driving along the road," I told him. "Muriel was behind me and said she saw flames coming out alarmingly. All I could hear was the awful noise. It was quite a dramatic journey back to the office from a patient's house!"

Later, I graduated from a Mini to a Metro. I was forever locking the door with the keys inside. One day Evelyn and I had parked our cars on a busy main road to visit a patient. When we came out I discovered that, once again, I couldn't get into my Metro. There were the keys inside and there was I on the outside.

"Oh, no, not again," I sighed. "I keep putting the keys down to pick up my bag, then I snib the lock without noticing they're still on the seat. Whatever will I do, we're late as it is."

"Hold on a cotton picking minute before you panic," said Evelyn, "I've got some of that reinforced paper you use for tying parcels. It's great for opening car doors. You're lucky you've got your Auntie Evelyn with you today."

So we stood in the street in our nurses' uniforms breaking into my car door with no trouble at all. Just then a man came up and went to his car parked next to mine. His was a Porsche.

"It's OK," Evelyn reassured him. "We haven't got as far as yours, we're still working our way up the street."

"We learnt this at the college as part of our course, so we're putting it into practice," I added. He looked at us darkly, jumped into the driving seat and roared off with little regard for the speed limit!

"We really got him worried then," Evelyn laughed. "Our next joint venture will be car theft. We'll be a lot richer then, that's for sure."

"I'm known to the police already, so I'd better opt out of that," I said.

"Jings, crivvens and help my kilt! I knew you'd be found out some day for speeding," Evelyn said.

"It wasn't for speeding it was for illegal parking! In fact it happened twice, but I only had to go to the police station once."

"This is getting worse by the minute. Never mind, I'll come and visit you when you're locked up in Craiginches."

"The first time it happened I hadn't long started on the district. I was on King Street. It was a blizzard of snow. I was carrying heaps of dressings packs into the house," I continued. "I'd already been round and round in circles, trying to find a place to park. I didn't want the packs to get soaked. So I parked at the door, half up on the pavement. I was upstairs washing my hands when I heard a stern voice. 'WHERE'S THE NURSE?' I turned round and nearly had a heart attack, there was this policeman at least ten feet tall blocking the bathroom door."

"You must have got a real scare. So what happened?" Evelyn asked.

"He said I was causing an obstruction, there were all these big lorries backed up along the road behind my wee car. But even so, he was very nice. He told me I could finish dressing the patient's wound, but not to let it happen again."

"So you were let off that time, but what about the next?"

"It was the Saturday before Christmas. I went to answer an emergency call from the Denburn Health Centre. When I came back the car park was heaving – all those Christmas shoppers. I drove back out into the street and parked outside a block of flats."

"Is that where those wee humpy things are – they prang your car if try to go over them," Evelyn said.

"Is that what they're for? When I came back at five o'clock, it was pitch dark. There was my Mini. It had been pushed further down the street and there was a pencilled note on pink paper stuck to my windscreen telling me I had to report to the police at Lodge Walk, 2 p.m. on Sunday afternoon."

"Jings, Margaret I was right about Craiginches. You're on the way there sure enough," Evelyn exclaimed.

"They took all my details including my mother's maiden name. But of course I was still on duty. They said they'd explain my situation to the man who'd reported me. It was him and the policeman who had lifted up my car and carried it down the street. I never heard any more about it so he must have decided not to take it any further."

"Your guardian angel has a hard time looking after you," Evelyn sighed.

"I was worried sick every time the postie stuck mail through our letter box in case it was my summons to the court."

"Life's a sair fecht at times indeed, Margaret," Evelyn said with a rueful laugh.

Parking was a major headache and grew worse as the time went on. Double yellow lines seemed to appear over night, and parking meters sprung up like mushrooms.

"I got a parking ticket today," Gail told us dolefully one lunchtime. " I thought my 'Nurse on Call' sticker would get me off a fine. What a hope!"

"Those stickers are a waste of time. The traffic wardens don't recognise them as genuine," Evelyn agreed.

"We're supposed to phone their office if we think we're going to have a problem with parking," I added. "Even so you can't park on yellow lines unless you're delivering some equipment"

"Dinna worry, Gail," Muriel consoled her, "I've kept a copy of the last letter I wrote to the Chief Constable asking to be let off. If you write to them in good time, you dinna hae to pay the fine. You can copy my letter."

So we kept a copy of Muriel's letter. We used it every time we had a parking summons.

"Where's that letter? I've had another ticket!" Gail said one day. "How do those wardens expect us to get round our patients? They'll be making us ride bikes next."

"My father-in-law in Lossiemouth discovered papers in beautiful copperplate handwriting describing the district nurse's working conditions almost a hundred years ago," I said. "Guess what, the nurse had to pay part rent on her bicycle. Some things never change!"

"Bike or car, nurses aye hae to finance the service we give, " Sheila agreed. "Did those old Lossie papers tell you anything aboot patient care? "

"They mention those dressings Muriel and I learnt about when we were students, jaconet and oiled silk. The only other equipment she carried was a Higginson's syringe."

"So she was giving enemas in those days. That work never changes either," Muriel remarked.

"The nurse was the only one in the town for years. She never married and the Lossie folk contributed to a house for her when she retired… By the way, talking about marriage, how are your wedding plans going, Sheila?" I asked.

"I'll be sending out the invitations next month," Sheila went on. "It'll be great to hae you crowd at my wedding."

"I'm sure some of our patients would like to see you in your wedding dress," I said.

"I've promised them a' I'll bring in the photos."

Just before the wedding, Gail and Evelyn got to work on the unsuspecting bride.

"We'll have a fashion show." Gail and Evelyn told Muriel and me. "We'll dress Sheila up."

They decorated Sheila with elastoplast and bandages, safety pins and paper clips, put her into one of the largest size nappy pads they could find, then suspended syringes and boxes of suppositories round her.

"Are ye nae deen yet?" Sheila protested, laughing, "I must look a richt feel like this."

"You stand still and keep quiet," Gail ordered. "We're not satisfied with you yet. What else can you find in the cupboard, Evelyn?"

"I've got an old nylon nightie for a veil, and look, here's a pillow to make her look nine months pregnant. We'll cover that with a plastic apron." Evelyn emerged from the cupboard with her arms full.

"You look a beautiful bride now, Sheila," Muriel and I joked. "Donnie would really fancy you in that outfit."

"Right, now it's time to show you off to the rest of the practice," Gail said.

Sheila was paraded around the staff coffee room. Then Gail and Evelyn drove her to some of her patients' homes. It brightened up the old folks' day and gave them something to laugh about for ages afterwards.

"Even aul Granny Leith gave a smile when she saw me," Sheila told us. "She asked for a wee drop of brandy to drink my health."

And so did we all on Sheila's wedding day.

Chapter 16: A place where you go on living right until the end

One of my diabetic patients whom I visited every day, Bob, was insulin dependent and also crippled with a hip injury that refused to heal. Bob lived with his wife Lily in a bungalow in a residential area.

One Monday morning, Muriel phoned me at home. She had been working that weekend and had done Bob's routine visits.

"Margaret, I ken you give Bob his insulin on your way into the practice. An affa' thing happened at the weekend," she said. "When I called on Saturday morning I was met with great clouds of smoke coming oot under their front door…"

"Oh, my goodness, don't tell me they've set their house on fire. Are they okay?"

"I had to hunt for them through a' the smoke. I finally found them soon' and roon' in the spare bedroom. Just then the fire brigade arrived and the story cam' oot," Muriel went on.

"We wis getting ready for oor bed when we saw the electric blanket wis on fire," Bob had said. "I telt Lily to go awa' oot the back and fill the rooser with water. She poored the water oot ower the bed, hauled up the covers and we went awa' ben the hoose for the nicht. We never thocht the flames would ging on smouldering the hale nicht."

"I can just see Lily trying to put out the flames with that old watering can just as if she was watering the roses," I laughed, relieved that the old couple were none the worse. "I expect they've gone to stay with their son to get away from the smoke."

"That's just the problem. Their son came roond and we baith tried to persuade them to flit up the road, but you ken Bob… "

"Weel, weel, nae langer or ae nicht," Bob had agreed reluctantly. "Lily and I are nae going awa oot o' this hoose till we're cairried oot in a box."

"So they're in their ain hame," Muriel went on, "but it's thick wi' reek. I dinna ken how they can bide there. I wis hoasting for the rest of the morning efter I left them."

"It was really bad in there, I felt I was being choked to death, the fumes were so thick, but the two of them won't budge from that house," I told Muriel in the afternoon.

"Aye I ken. I still canna believe that they're alive. Their aul fashioned furniture must have saved them. Modern stuff would hae given off worse fumes. I never want to come across a thing like that again, that's for sure. I was fleggit to death when I saw a' the reek coming under the door."

Eventually they agreed to have the house redecorated. But even then they wouldn't move.

"Ilka ane's as thrawn as the ither," their son said despairingly.

"They'll do their own thing no matter what," I agreed. "That's what keeps them going."

Palliative care now became a discipline in its own right. District nurses were invited to spend a day in the local hospice, Roxburghe House, learning about the principles of pain relief and symptom control for terminally ill patients.

I was so impressed with the peaceful atmosphere and the high standard of nursing care that I told my colleagues, "Everybody thinks that a hospice is where you go to die. It's not: it's a place where you go on living right until the end."

Six months later, my nurse manager gave me the opportunity to develop a liaison service between the hospice and the community. Roxburghe House operates an open door policy. Patients whose symptoms had been brought under control returned home, knowing that there would always be a bed for them in the hospice the moment it was needed. My role was to facilitate admission and discharge plans for patients in the hospice as well as those in the wider community, while still continuing to work with my usual caseload on the district.

I appreciated the co-operation of my colleagues to enable me to undertake this new venture.

"It helps us too," Sheila assured me. "You bring us up to date with all the latest techniques for terminal care. I feel much more confident about counselling now I've done that course you told me about."

"Mind Mr Smith with bone cancer?" Muriel said. "They did so much to relieve his pain in Roxburghe, he was back driving his car and working in his gairden. It wasna just the drugs, but the way he got hope and encouragement there that gave him a new lease of life."

"That's what the hospice is all about," I replied.

Princess Diana once paid a visit to Roxburghe House. I arrived in the hospice later that day to find the whole place buzzing with the news of the royal occasion. People were thrilled and everyone praised the Princess so highly. She sat beside each patient and talked to them, undeterred by the fact some of them were so near death. One lady had told the Princess, "You're talking to somebody who is the same age as the Queen Mother." The old lady died that same night.

The hospice receptionist, nurses and doctors were all welcoming and supportive whenever I came. Little did I know then that one pretty, efficient young nurse would become my daughter-in-law. I would have enjoyed my time there even more if I'd had a crystal ball to see into the future!

The patients and staff in the hospice together took away the fear and foreboding of cancer. The whole concept of hospice work is to enhance the quality of life remaining to the patients and their families wherever they chose to be, either in their own homes or in the hospice. People were encouraged to express their worries; families were involved in each stage of the dying process. Cancer had been the great unspoken taboo. It was wonderful to see the changes that understanding and honesty brought.

In order to extend my knowledge of pain and symptom control for patients at home, I attended a cancer care course. Pain control was becoming easier to manage at home, especially with syringe drivers to deliver opiates at a continuous rate. The correct dosage of the drug, usually heroin, was given continuously over a twenty-four hour period. Patients could hope for a better night's sleep and no longer had to worry in case the nurse was delayed in coming to give an injection every four hours day and night. Nursing cancer patients at home is a privilege, and the mutual support that grew between nurses and families meant that bereavement follow up also became a meaningful part of our work. As drug therapy for terminal illness improved we found that our GP colleagues and ourselves really became a partnership in care giving.

George was in his early forties when he developed terminal prostate cancer. His mother had died the year before after having a stroke, and he lived with his father and his sister, Iris. George had cerebral palsy, so communication with him was extremely difficult. Sheila and Gail were both involved in George's care.

"George is dying, Margaret, and his sister Iris is nae really coping." Sheila told me one day. "She's exhausted. George is a clever lad and kens fit's going on, but he canna talk. Iris can mak him oot, but everybody else has problems. He's scared wi' the idea of hospitals. Iris says she darena' mention the hospice."

"What do you think we can do to help them?" I asked.

"I was wondering if there was a way of getting money from the Macmillan Fund for him to hae round the clock nursing care at hame," Sheila said.

"That's a great idea, Sheila," I replied. "I'll speak to Doctor Ingram when I'm out at Roxburghe tomorrow and see what he can do."

Dr. Ingram, the consultant from the hospice visited George at home and arranged to fund nurses to stay with him all the time. George died peacefully at home. Iris had him laid out dressed in an ordinary jersey and trousers, and he lay on the settee in the living room until the day of the funeral, still a much loved member of the family.

We continued to care for this family as George's father then developed Alzheimer's Disease. Iris looked after him too, despite his increasing confusion. Gail and Iris became great friends over the years. Iris too developed cancer, small reward after all her years of caring.

Husbands cared for wives, wives for husbands. Children too helped in the caring. Family support is essential if somebody with a terminal illness is nursed at home. You can see then which families are strong and caring of one another. The courage and love we saw in difficult circumstances helped us in our work.

One family's commitment and care of one of their own was wonderful and humbling to see. They were a family of six. The mother, Joan and father, Neil had three daughters, Kathleen, Dawn and Michelle, and a son called John.

The first of their troubles came when Michelle was nine years. She was playing on the pavement outside her home when a van driver careered into her. Michelle was rushed to hospital and her right foot was amputated. The next year Dawn started to become unwell. She was fifteen, and at first her irrational behaviour was put down to teenage rebellion, but soon her condition deteriorated to the extent that she became utterly helpless. Dawn had developed a syndrome called encepalopathy. It was attributed to the measles virus reactivating itself.

At present there is great debate about the safety of the triple vaccine for measles, mumps and rubella. Parents are concerned about its link with autism and inflammatory bowel disease. A measles epidemic is now feared to be possible because of the low uptake of the vaccination. The long-term damage the measles virus caused to Dawn is the other side of the argument about vaccination. There are no easy answers in this dilemma.

The family visited Dawn every day in the hospital, but Michelle was still facing more surgery: her stump needed to be refashioned as she grew older.

"We'll take Dawn home and look after her," they decided.

"You'll never manage to look after Dawn yourselves. She's totally dependent, she needs professional nursing care," the hospital doctor warned.

"We'll have a good try," the parents replied. "We'll speak to our GP and ask for a district nurse."

Muriel was the nurse who helped them to care for Dawn. She built up a great relationship with all the family.

"That family are fantastic," Muriel told us. "Dawn's bed is in the living room. She's never left alone. Her Mum and Dad sleep on a bed settee beside her. There's a great big poster of Elvis on the wall, and they play a' her favourite pop songs. They put her in her wheelchair, tak' her oot in the car, and do everything wi' her."

"Do you think Dawn's aware of them even though she's completely unresponsive to everyone else?" I asked. "I feel she knows it's somebody strange when I'm there instead of you."

"I'm sure she kens them, though maybe nae so much as they would like to think, but she's aye mair relaxed wi' her mum or her sisters in the room," Muriel said.

Kathleen and the mother Joan were the ones who did most of the care, which included feeding Dawn through a tube in her stomach, and preventing her from developing pressure sores. Despite being a redhead with the fair skin that goes with it, Dawn's skin stayed intact, a tribute to the way she was turned and repositioned, day and night.

"I'm sure if Dawn had stayed in hospital she would have got a pressure sore by now," I said to Muriel.

"Aye, it's strange the way folk at hame never get the sores they do in the hospital. I've often wondered if the starch on the hospital sheets is bad for their skin," Muriel mused.

"Mind you, Dawn's weel nourished wi' her gastrostomy feeds, that maks a difference too."

"She was quite wee and slim when she first came home, now she seems taller and heavier each time I see her," I replied.

Dawn died of a chest infection when she was twenty-two. I was with her at the time as Muriel had a day off, and the doctor was also there, writing out a prescription for more antibiotics. Her mother Joan was so determined to give Dawn every chance. She had been through so many urinary and chest infections and they had always managed to pull her through before.

Kathleen and Michelle had both had babies during the years of Dawn's illness, so there were little toddlers crawling about as their young mothers washed Dawn and dressed her in the latest fashions. The little ones grew from newborn babies and her brother John moved from primary to secondary school while Dawn lay in her strange limbo. She still had her beautiful red hair, but her limbs had contracted and her muscles were wasted after six years of total unconsciousness.

Dawn had been terminally ill, although not with cancer. However, when terminal care is spoken about, cancer is the illness that springs to mind, with all the pain and distress associated with it. My liaison work with the hospice enabled me to take part in workshops, along with the doctor and sister in charge of the hospice, for the benefit of community nurses throughout the Grampian Region.

"You know I really enjoy teaching nurses about terminal care, but I know my teaching skills could be improved," I said. "How would you ones manage if I did the practical work teachers' course? It's a six-week course in blocks of two weeks at a time so I wouldn't be away at the college for too long at a time."

"You go ahead, Margaret. It'll help us in the long run because you'll have district nurse students working here once you're qualified," Muriel encouraged me.

The college ran courses for social work students, health care workers and offshore survival training, mandatory for all workers on the oil rigs. We were a strange mix when we met in the canteen! Trendy social work students mingled with big hulky men in jeans and anoraks. Then there were us, a small group of health visitors and district nurses in our thirties and forties.

Once again, as in the District Nursing course, nurses came to the college in Aberdeen from the Highlands and Islands to develop their skills to become practical work teachers. I got a great surprise, because one of the district nurses was Sally, my old friend from all those years ago in Glasgow Royal.

"How marvellous to see you again, Margaret!" She greeted me with a big hug.

"It's great to see you, Sally. I heard you'd moved from Lewis but that wasn't yesterday."

"I'm still living in Shetland. Roddy's never been shifted south, so I've kept on with my nursing there."

"Come and stay with us at the weekend," I invited. "We can phone Carol and have a chat."

"That'll be great, we'll catch up on old times. It'll be fine to see your David again," Sally said. "I'm glad now I agreed to go on this course. I wasn't keen, but my manager put a bit of pressure on for me to do it."

"Sally, I can't tell you how much seeing you again has boosted me up. I came here this morning feeling very sad – my oldest son, James left home last night. He's emigrated to South Africa. It's a great opportunity for him, but it's left me very down in the dumps. Goodness knows when I'll see him again. You've cheered me up no end."

"I know how you feel, Margaret, because my oldest boy has just gone away to join the Army, so I've been through the same thing."

"We'll keep each other going, just like we did in the old days in the Royal when things got on top of us," I said.

"There's no friends like old friends," Sally agreed.

I phoned Carol that night, and she came up to Aberdeen for a grand reunion.

Carol told us that she hadn't managed to go back to full time work because of her husband's work commitments.

"I'm keeping my hand in, though," she said. "I'm doing a research project for the GPs in Montrose."

"That sounds interesting, what are you researching?" we asked.

"I'm looking at patients with heart disease, to evaluate if exercise and diet prevent them needing to take heaps of heart pills. The Government aims to reduce heart disease in Scotland. It's potentially a big project."

So we caught up with all the news and discovered that none of us had heard from Joan.

"It's so easy to lose touch," we agreed and promised we three would do our best to keep in contact.

"You'll have to brave the wild sea and come up to Shetland for a holiday both of you." Sally said.

* * *

Now I had qualified as a practical work teacher I gave lectures on the practical aspects of palliative nursing care to district nurse students in the college. It was a great privilege to pass on knowledge that would help these nurses to manage terminal care in the community.

My links with the college continued after it had become a university. I was asked to be a member of the committee set up to develop community nursing as a degree course. This gave me an insight into the academic world

It was a long way from my student days of sitting in a classroom wearing starched dress, collar and cap, listening to nurse tutors talking about anatomy and bandaging! It was also a different world from my workaday one of leg ulcer dressings, injections, catheter and wound care, terminal care, and a variety of other things, not forgetting the giving of enemas.

"I went to a meeting at the university this morning," I said to Muriel one afternoon.

"Were you nae too busy, how did you fit it a' in?" she asked.

"Och well, I started work early in the morning. But I went into the meeting with all these lecturers and professors, having spent nearly an hour giving Mr Jones an enema. I thought, 'have I come from the sublime to the ridiculous or is it the other way round!'"

So I was now a practical work teacher of students studying for a diploma in district nursing. I remembered how much I'd learnt from Liz when I was a student. She'd seemed so experienced to me! I think I was as nervous as my first student when we started working together. She was called Wendy, and was very talented at drawing cartoons.

One day I was so earnestly explaining the situation in the home we'd just left, and why I'd given the care, that I drove up a one way street the wrong way. Wendy drew a cartoon of herself with her hair standing on end, three fags in her mouth, a bottle of valium and a bottle of whisky beside her. The caption read, "I see you've been out in the car with Margaret again!"

Evelyn agreed with the sentiments. "That picture's going up on the wall! Don't you dare to take it down," she told me severely.

"OK, OBE." I agreed meekly.

The patients liked having student nurses. They enjoyed having medical students too. One medical student helped dig my car out of a snow-drift when I was totally stuck – he was definitely worth having around!

Muriel, Sheila and I also felt that students enhanced our work with their forward thinking. No longer were young nurses afraid to express an opinion or challenge old-fashioned ideas and practices; we were glad to share in discussions about the reasons for giving care in a certain way.

"You young anes fairly keep us up to date wi' a' the latest ideas," Muriel told Wendy.

"Ah, but us oldies can still show you a few tricks," Evelyn said.

"Especially when it comes to car theft," I reminded her with a laugh.

Chapter 17: Booze, Buns and Bubbles

Muriel visited a confused old lady whose nephew was in charge of her money; unfortunately he had a drink problem, and that used up Auntie's money too.

"I feel so sorry for Mrs Dalgarno, there's nae food at a' in the hoose. I'll refer her to the social worker," Muriel told Sheila and me.

"I know you go to the shops to buy a bite of dinner for her yourself, Muriel, I saw you going into her house the other day with a bag of messages," I said.

"Weel, it's better than the aul wife nae haeing a bittie denner. I canna ging hame to eat and think of her wi' nae food."

The social worker came to assess the situation.

"There was a pot boiling on the stove. She was obviously preparing something for lunch," she reported back to Muriel.

"But did you nae look inside the pot?" Muriel replied, "It's her vest and knickers she's got cooking in there!"

Appearances are always deceptive, and Mrs Beattie too proved the point. She was a lady with a drink problem. As a young staff nurse I hadn't realised that well-spoken ladies living in respectable areas of the town could knock back the booze, but now I knew not to be fooled by pleasant exteriors, both of people and buildings!

"Mrs Beattie refuses to go to bed, she sits up all night drinking her gin," Evelyn told me in an exasperated voice. "I threaten her with a good skelping if she hasn't slept in her bed, but help my kilt, next morning she's still sitting there in that armchair."

"I know, she's got terrible swollen legs and they've been cut to pieces with all the falls she has," I agreed. "You try to keep her clean and I try to heal her sores and neither of us is winning. Besides, the place stinks with the cats."

Mrs Beattie was very fond of cats. She would phone the Cat

Protection League and take in strays. The cats were incontinent and so was she.

She was such a pleasant lady, but it was an impossible situation, made worse when her daughter, Marie, who also had a drink problem, came to live with her. One Hogmanay, I called to dress the cuts on Mrs Beattie's legs. It was 5 p.m. and I knew that if I didn't gain access to the house, there would be no dressings done till after the holiday period was over. The doorbell didn't work, so I shouted through the letterbox, "Please let me in!"

Eventually Marie lurched to the door with a glass of whisky in her hand.

"There's somebody for you, Mummy dear," she said, and staggered past the door and up the stairs. Outside it was a beautiful frosty night, the last streaks of a sunset were in the sky, and the stars were appearing. Owls were hooting in the nearby wood.

At last, Mrs Beattie struggled to the door and let me in. In the kitchen some broken glasses lay on the floor. On the table in the living room the cat was enjoying the remains of a Chinese carry-out.

"Mrs Beattie had already obviously started to celebrate Hogmanay a few hours early. I ignored the mess everywhere, dressed her ulcers, wished her a happy New Year and went home," I told Evelyn once we were all back at work after the holiday break.

"It would be just the same New Year or not," Evelyn said philosophically. "I emptied out her glass of gin today, mistaking it for water that had been lying around all night. She got all huffy with me, but I sang 'Campbelltown Loch I wish you were whisky' and we parted good friends."

Once Evelyn visited Mrs Beattie and found her semiconscious. She phoned me at the practice and I rushed up. The ambulance men arrived on the scene just after, and our patient was admitted to hospital where she spent several weeks drying out. While her mother was in hospital, Marie was "fostered" by a lady who took in people recovering from alcohol abuse. Marie was helped to overcome her addiction and was given a flat on her own, although she had several relapses. Evelyn always kept in touch, and popped in to see her when she was in the vicinity.

One day, Evelyn and I were back at the surgery at the end of our morning's work, planning the visits for the next day when the receptionist phoned:

"There's somebody collapsed in the office across the road. They've phoned here, but the doctors are out on their rounds or busy in the surgery. Can you help?"

We rushed across the road and up three flights of stairs to find a man in his forties lying in the recovery position. One of his colleagues knew a bit of first aid, but in spite of his efforts his friend had stopped breathing. Evelyn and I started doing cardiopulmonary resuscitation, thankful that we were given regular practice to keep up our skills. We managed to start him breathing again, and then the paramedics arrived. They were brilliant in their handling of the situation. Our patient had to be carried down the three flights of stairs we'd raced up a short time before. He arrested again but the paramedics had the necessary drugs on hand to bring him around. They took him to hospital, where unfortunately he couldn't be saved. We heard later that he'd died from a massive brain haemorrhage.

"I'm still out of breath from those stairs," Evelyn told Gail. "I thought Margaret would be under a bus, she raced across the road so fast, and she was up those stairs in a flash. All I could see was a glimpse of blue away ahead of me."

"Well, you *are* ten years older than Margaret," Gail consoled her. "You did OK you know."

"Thanks for reminding me," Evelyn remarked. "But I tell you, even though her new name *is* McColgan, I stopped Margaret in her tracks our last weekend on. She couldn't move so fast then."

"She left me suspended in thin air," I told Gail. "Our OBE stuck me in a hoist in a patient's house. 'I'm just showing the nurse how it works,' she said to the lady. Then she pushed the old wifie in her wheelchair through to her living room. I was helpless till she came back for me."

"At least she didn't have a cup of coffee first," Gail said to me. "I wouldn't put it past her."

"Nor would I," I agreed. "I would have had to call out, ' Help, where's the nurse?' "

* * *

"I'm in despair trying to treat Rose's leg ulcers," I said one day in the office.

Rose had lived with her parents, and after they died she stayed on in the house alone. She had few friends or close relatives. Rose once drove a car, but she was housebound now. She told me that she used to take her parents out in the car for their shopping. She had never learnt how to reverse, so she drove out to Banchory to the butcher's to save her from having to manoeuvre the car into a parking place in Aberdeen.

Rose was typical of a lonely patient with leg ulcers. She enjoyed the company of the nurses and didn't really want her legs to heal. In her case she made matters worse because she sat up all night; her arthritis was too painful for her to get in and out of bed. She didn't sit with her legs up during the day, and she didn't cook proper meals. I tried to persuade her to buy fish from a fish van to improve her diet, in the hope that better food would promote healing. The man came round the doors delivering beautiful fresh fish from the Moray Firth. Rose got quite excited by this idea, but it ended up with her buying the tasty scones and cakes he also sold.

I would come into her kitchen and say, "Did you get a nice piece of lemon sole today, Rose?"

"No, he had such fine iced buns, I thought I'd treat myself to them instead," she replied rather guiltily.

I brought her in some of my turkey and Christmas pudding when

I worked over the Christmas period, to give her a share of festive cheer. She had to have her legs dressed even on Christmas Day and if I were on duty, I would arrange to visit her myself. We pooled the work amongst the nurses, but we all preferred to visit the patients "on our books" rather than ones we didn't know, and of course they wanted their "own" nurse too.

"Where's my ain nurse?" some of the old folk would say. "I dinna ken fa you are."

"You've been going to Rose all these years, Margaret," Muriel remarked. "And that wee lassie with the motor scooter, Sarah had her before you. And I still go to Minnie."

"Yes, she's another one we inherited from Sarah," I said.

"Minnie aye gies us an apple or an orange," Muriel said. "If she had eaten the fruit herself her leg might have healed by now! 'Here's your aipplie my dearie, dinna forget it noo,' she says when we try to leave withoot it."

The fruit shop must have been pleased when Minnie's legs needed attention.

Her ulcers would occasionally heal over for a month or two, but they broke down again with great regularity. We enjoyed visiting her as much as she liked our visits. Minnie had been brought up in the little fishing village at Aberdeen harbour. She had a great fund of stories. She remembered the man coming round the doors selling dulse or edible seaweed, for the children.

"There wasna ice cream for the bairnies then," she said, "But we likit the dulse fine."

It was probably a lot better for their teeth!

During the war, Minnie had done a man's work in the shipyards in Belfast as well as Aberdeen. She recalled that eating dry oatcakes was a great cure for seasickness.

"A'body was seek but me," she reminisced. "I had my oatcakes and I had nae bother at a'."

Another patient also with arthritis and legs that wouldn't heal was

Father O'Connor. In his retirement he was cared for by nuns in the Catholic home for the elderly.

"Sister Theresa says Father O'Connor bosses the nuns about. They're thankful it's us nurses who are called in to do his legs," I said to Muriel. "He's such an old curmudgeon he won't co-operate."

"Aye, I ken. He says he canna put his legs up at a'. It taks me at least forty-five minutes to try to get at all the bitties of ulcers at the back of his legs. "

"All that kneeling to get at all the sore bits is not good for the knees. I've got district nurse's knee, not housemaid's knee," I agreed.

Father O'Connor had been a teacher at a boys' boarding school in a remote area of the Highlands. He used to tell us about the wonderful colours of the Northern Lights on winter nights.

"I've got Father O'Connor a half bottle of whisky for his Christmas, Margaret. He hasna got family to buy him presents," Muriel told me.

"I thought of that too," I said. "I've got him a book of meditation by Thomas a Kempis. I suppose we're each giving him spiritual gifts, but I bet he enjoys yours the most!"

"Talking about Christmas, are you going to the practice night out?" I asked.

"Aye, I'm looking forward to it. Mind last year? The ceilidh band was great."

"I'm going to make sure we all dance 'Strip the Willow'," Evelyn said.

The Friday afternoon of the night out came the phone call we all dreaded, "Mr Dick is constipated. Please could you call to give an enema?"

"It's always the same!" I sighed. "They wait all week and decide on Friday they'd better call the doctor, who then summons us. I bet Mr Dick's been taking codeine with the usual results. I'll go and sort him out," I volunteered.

So off I went armed with the rubber tubing and funnel we used to give a soap and water enema.

"Fairy Liquid usually works," I thought as I drove across the city.

"That ad about soft hands doesn't proclaim all the benefits of this dish washing liquid."

Unfortunately Mrs Dick had the special offer economy variety of washing up liquid with very poor results as far as the long-suffering patient was concerned. I was getting stressed out too. It was by now five thirty and I thought about the dinner that was ahead of me. I was running out of time to put on the glamour!

I asked Mrs Dick if she had any stronger liquid cleaner.

"Fit aboot this, nursie, will it dee?" She delved into her cupboard and brought out a bottle of "Jif" bathroom cleaner.

"Well no, I don't think we'd better use that. I hate to think what your husband's insides would be like after a dose of Jif, we'll just have to carry on with what we've got."

Eventually there was a happy conclusion, and I drove home to soak in a bath filled with nice scented bubbles.

"Perhaps I should have poured bubble bath down that funnel instead," I thought before disappearing into the foam.

* * *

Some of the men we visited were very keen gardeners. Several had been farmers or farm workers. They would give us bags of potatoes or a cabbage, or cuttings from their begonias.

"When you go to Mrs Angus, you have to be sure to give her husband Wullie the used colostomy and urine drainage bags," Evelyn remarked over a cup of coffee in the office.

"I ken, he aye stands at the foot of the bed watching a' we're deeing," Sheila replied. "'Dinna teem those oot, gie them ower tae me,' he says, and then he taks the bags awa wrapped up in newspaper so we canna see fit he's deeing wi' them."

"I'm sure that's why his roses win prizes in all the competitions," Evelyn said.

"Aul Jimmy's anither fa wants to win the prize when Aberdeen is competing for the Britain in Bloom award," Sheila went on. "He's got the bonniest gairden, wi' flooers he's grown from seed and from cuttings. It's a treat to walk up his path and stand at the door, smelling a' the fine scent."

"The bathroom's full of seedlings in little pots. Even the bath's full of plants. It's just as well Jimmy and Aggie never ask us to give them a bath," Evelyn laughed.

For other people it was the house rather than the garden that took up their attention.

A lady called Irene was always having alterations done to her house. She lived with her diabetic husband. Diabetic patients who needed insulin injections were always the first to be visited each day. Sandy was one of my patients. He needed insulin twice a day. Irene also had medical problems, ranging from arthritis to diverticulitis, which eventually resulted in her having a colostomy.

"Irene's always calling out the doctor for herself, and for Sandy, and the vet for the cat and the dog," I said to my student Wendy on her next time out from the college. "I'm glad to see you back for your second practical experience. You can take over their care for me. You have to have a diabetic patient as part of your caseload."

"I'll be glad to do that, Margaret, "Wendy replied. "I know I've got a challenge ahead of me with Irene. The cupboard's full of sweeties," Wendy continued, "I keep telling Irene that Sandy shouldn't have them but she doesn't listen. By the way, her house is beautiful isn't it? She's got a real gift for interior design."

"I was forever stepping over joiners and painters when I first went there," I remembered. "Irene loved home decorating so much she always drove Sandy and the little dog for miles out in the country to visit antique shops. She kept trying to match the wallpaper or the curtains with a lampshade or an ornament to bring out a certain shade. Irene's certainly very talented, but she drove me up the wall because they would be late back for Sandy's afternoon injection. She always had me waiting on the doorstep for ages. "

I would be waiting outside fuming because it was late and I should have been finished work an hour before. Then I would see the car coming about ten miles an hour along the road, Irene driving with Sandy sitting beside her and Roy the dog perched on his knee. Sandy would be so pleased with his outing and Irene so pleased with her latest acquisition that I couldn't let on how annoyed I felt.

As they grew frailer they employed a home help privately.

"Jan, the home help is so good to them. Even a daughter wouldn't do as much as she does," Wendy observed.

"I know, she's really special," I agreed.

"I'll be back in the college next week," Wendy told me. "I've learnt so much with you, Margaret, it's been a great time."

"I've enjoyed teaching you, Wendy," I replied. " I'll be at a meeting with you and your tutors whilst you're back for your next lot of lectures. I'll see you again then, and I'm looking forward to it for myself too, because my friend Sally will probably be down from Shetland."

So I met Sally again back in the college.

"You've never managed up to Shetland to visit us," Sally remarked.

"It's because I have a grandson in South Africa now. James got married to a lovely girl out there. So I save up all my holidays to go to see them."

"Well, it's a lot warmer than Lerwick, that's for sure," Sally agreed.

"My son's been home on leave from the army, he's really grown up in a short time," Sally continued. "When he complains about the sergeant major shouting at him, I tell him about those sisters who used to bawl us out. 'We were treated as though we were in the army too,' I tell him."

"So we were," I said ruefully, "By the way I heard from Carol, her daughter's planning a wedding next year, so that's something to look forward to. It's amazing how the time passes isn't it?" I went on. "It doesn't seem long since we were all getting engaged and married ourselves."

"Well, Margaret that's a real sign of old age," Sally teased me. "You sound just like some of those old folks we look after."

"I am a granny after all," I said. And with that we went in to a meeting with our students.

Chapter 18: Community Cares?

During the Thatcherite years, politics brought changes to the management of nursing care. Our organisation became a health care trust. We were providers of care, but the social services and the general practitioners were the purchasers. The social services began to take on the role of home carers, doing basic tasks of personal hygiene that had been performed by community nurses. There was a charge for their care packages whereas our care was given free.

Our nursing management went through change after change, and the paperwork piled up with each change. We now had to fill in forms to refer people for services that we'd already assessed they needed. A social worker then went out and reassessed them, so why had we bothered in the first place?

Our uniform was changed from dresses to trousers, from Harris tweed coats to working men's jackets.

"I feel really worried about what will happen to the Harris tweed industry, now they haven't got the order for our coats," I commented when we wore our new uniforms.

"These trousers are such a hideous turquoise colour. Some of the patients are calling us Smurfs," Gail added.

"I like the jacket, it's easier to wear in the car," Muriel tried to be positive. "But the bright blue breeks dinna go wi' the navy jacket at a'. Mind Snuffy Ivy's lime green breeks? These are almost as bright!"

"It's the corporate image, so that we match the logo of the Trust. It's so corporate that it's only the female nurses who are forced to wear it," I complained. "If the men did too, we would know they really meant it."

"It doesna look so bad in the hospital," Sheila said. "The nurses wear the white tunic and that goes better wi' the breeks, but they look really loud against the navy jacket."

"One lady asked if I was the postie when she saw my big jacket," Evelyn added. "Nobody knows we're nurses now."

The general consensus was that the new uniform was a big clanger on the part of the senior management, who certainly weren't the ones who had to parade the streets in this gear.

One manager we had for a short time had been a health visitor before moving into management. Geoffrey seemed to understand the changes we found so bewildering.

"We're going to do a SWOT analysis," he announced one day.

"Whatever's that?" we wondered. "Swot was a word we used at school," we told each other.

"SWOT or nae SWOT, I need Geoffrey's advice," Sheila told us. "I'm expecting a baby and I want to arrange to job share after my maternity leave."

Muriel and I congratulated her on her news. "You'll hae to be careful and nae do any heavy lifting," Muriel warned her.

"How are you keeping, Sheila?" I asked.

"I'm fine, I've nae morning sickness at a'. It's the running to the loo that's a problem," she said ruefully.

"You'll have to be like Evelyn and book the loos you fancy," I said. "I'm sure she organises her patients' visits round her favourite conveniences!"

"Geoffrey will help you arrange a job share. Mind, you'll hae to find someone we all get on wi'," Muriel said.

Linda joined our nursing team. She was a young mum, who had just returned to work after maternity leave. Linda was tall and slim with dark curly hair.

Linda and Sheila worked a week about. They were both very committed to making the job share work.

"We have the same ideas, and keep each other up to date, so the patients get continuity of care," Linda told me.

"Muriel and I both think it's working out really well," I reassured her. "In fact you're so in tune with each other, I think we'll call you either Sheilin or Linshei!"

"The patients never seem to mix you up. They aye ken fit ane o' you was in to see them, and they like to hear a' the stories you tell them of your babies, " Muriel said. "It fairly gies them something to speak aboot."

Then we were allocated another manager who didn't like the set up at all.

"Whoever heard of two nurses working a week about? That's not a proper job share. The other nurses in your position work two and a half days a week each," she complained to Sheila and Linda.

"Geoffrey organised this for us, and it works in with our caseload as well as with our families," they replied.

But it remained a source of contention between the management and our nursing team. Each change of manager seemed to make our relationship with them deteriorate further.

"You team of nurses are always uncooperative. I've heard all of you complain about the new uniform with those nice turquoise trousers, and it's been noted how you object to filling in the new computerised daily visit forms. But you'll have to agree to this latest decision. We want the auxiliary nurses to pool all their work amongst the various health centres. It makes more economic sense," we were told.

"That's it, I'm leaving. We're a good team here. I don't want to go to different patients every day. I'd spend all my time getting lost anyway," Evelyn was in great distress.

"I can't see the point in this either, and all the old folks will be asking us, 'Where's our OBE? they'll say'. If you and Gail get moved they'll be very upset." I agreed. "We'll have a meeting with the GPs. They won't be happy if you two aren't part of our nursing team either."

So we had a very acrimonious meeting with the doctors, the managers and ourselves. The upshot was that Gail and Evelyn stayed in our team to the mutual satisfaction of our patients, our doctor colleagues and ourselves.

Whilst we were having all these battles with management our

nursing commitments became ever more time consuming. Patients were being nursed at home with complex needs.

My student Wendy joined us from college for her final period of practical experience before her examination to gain a diploma in District Nursing.

"We're seeing people discharged home from hospital requiring complicated wound care," I explained to her. "We also have people on chemotherapy pumps, gastrostomy feeding tubes, more syringe drivers for giving pain and nausea relief in terminal care, even patients on ventilators to maintain their breathing."

"I was glad you were with me when we went to that new patient, Mrs Chapman yesterday. I hadn't ever cared for a patient with a Hickman line for giving chemotherapy. But now I've seen the way you do her dressing, I'm looking forward to having her on my caseload," Wendy told me as we were driving to visit this patient.

"Yes, Alison Chapman's a wonderful patient – she's always so brave. She's told me how much her church means to her now she's so ill. She really lives out her faith in her life," I replied. "In hospital she used to help to feed some of the old ladies in the ward, even though she was feeling so sick herself. She's had so much chemotherapy, yet her cancer keeps spreading."

"She's pleased we're so meticulous with our aseptic technique," Wendy said. "When you were in the bathroom washing your hands she said to me that all the nurses in the hospital are really particular about keeping her line sterile. But she added that the doctor came in to the ward last time she was there. He came to take blood from her line, and you'll never believe this, Margaret, he didn't wash his hands."

"I think some hospital doctors should spend time with the infection control nurse. It might cut down the number of hospital acquired infections," I agreed with Wendy.

"Mrs Chapman told me that she asked him to go and wash his hands," Wendy went on. "She said that once upon a time she would never have dared to tell a doctor what to do, but she's fighting to keep the cancer at bay and she's immuno-suppressed with all that chemotherapy."

"Good for her," I applauded. "She knows an infection in her line could kill her. But here we are at Alison Chapman's. Let's go in."

"Hello, there, how are you doing today, Alison?" I asked.

"I'm just fine. Hello Wendy, you're back again then?" Alison replied.

"Wendy's going to come to you regularly now, Alison. I'll pop in once a week to see how things are going," I said.

"That's perfectly all right, Wendy and I will get on fine together, won't we?" Alison smiled at Wendy.

"I cared for a little girl having chemotherapy two years ago," I told Wendy when we left Alison's house. "Angela was only nine, so she went to the Sick Kids' Hospital for all her treatment, but she learned how to care for her Hickman line herself. There are nurses there who teach the children. I used to bring in the equipment she needed and give the family support."

"How did she come on with the treatment?" Wendy wanted to know.

"She did really well. She had a non-Hodgkin's lymphoma and responded well to the chemotherapy. But she has a little brother, Luke and he was diagnosed with muscular dystrophy. What a burden some families have to bear!"

"That's terrible, because there's no treatment for that. It's a genetic thing isn't it?" Wendy said.

"Yes, and then their mother discovered she was expecting twins," I went on. "The family are devout Catholics so she wouldn't consider having the babies tested before they were born. She was worried she'd be pressurised into having a termination. So she had her twins, a little boy and a little girl, then they were tested to see if they would be affected too."

"It's the boy who's a risk with the girl likely to be a carrier isn't it?" Wendy asked

"Yes, but happily they were both all right. They moved down to England so I don't know how little Luke is, but the last time I saw Angela she looked great. She'd grown bigger, and her hair had come in beautifully thick and curly, because of course when I was visiting her it had all come out."

Wendy and I also cared for a lady with motor neurone disease. She had lost the ability to speak and swallow. We went up to the hospital to meet Mrs Duthie and her husband, so that when she came home they would feel more confident that she would get the help she needed.

"We'll ask the evening nurses to fix you up to the pump for your overnight tube feed," I assured them.

"My hands are too twisted with arthritis to manage to join the tube on to the bottles and set the pump," Mr Duthie said. "And Barbara of course hasna got the strength."

"We'll visit them every day to begin with. We may be able to reduce the number of visits in the week once they settle down," I said to Wendy.

"I'll find that hard when I'm qualified and working on my own, knowing when to withdraw. I would worry about folk who are so ill all the time," Wendy said.

"That's exactly what I said to my practical work teacher too," I recalled. "It's the hardest thing to do, but you have to make sure you've done all you can, and given them all the emergency numbers to call if necessary."

"That's all very well, but Barbara Duthie can't speak," Wendy pointed out. "If anything happened to Mr Duthie what on earth would she do?"

"I know it's a big problem, but they've got a son who lives nearby. He often pops in and I'm sure he'd take more to do with his mum if he had to," I reassured her.

Mrs Duthie also had epilepsy.

"Barbara's been free of fits for years because she always takes her medication regularly, but they've started up again," Mr Duthie told me worriedly.

"I think it's because she's not able to swallow her drugs properly even though you're giving them in liquid form," I said. "We'll have to start giving them to her down her tube. Wendy or I will do them first thing in the morning and again in the afternoon, and the evening nurses will do the last dose."

"Oh, Margaret, I'm so grateful for all your help," Mr Duthie said with relief.

"That's what we're here for," I replied. "It's a privilege for us to be able to help you and Mrs Duthie. You told me you served in the army during the war, and Mrs Duthie was in the WRNs; you've certainly done your best when you had to."

"That's true enough, I suppose," he agreed. "I just count my blessings that I survived when so many of my friends were lost. I was sent to India in the war, but the other regiment went to Singapore. They were all taken prisoner by the Japanese. I could so easily have died in a Japanese prison camp if my name had been on a different order sheet."

Our communication with Barbara was in writing. She had laboriously to write everything down in notepads. She still had the use of her arms even though they were growing weaker.

Wendy and I shared the visits until it was time for her to go back into college.

"I'll miss all these patients. You'll have to let me know how they get on," Wendy told me.

Both Alison and Barbara died at home within a short time of our conversation.

I went back to studying, too, this time to do a nurse prescribing course. Now I could prescribe various dressings, creams and lotions for my patients, but perhaps best of all nurses could write prescriptions for laxatives!

"No more enemas because people have been given codeine to take,"

I said to Muriel once I'd completed the course. "I'll make sure they all have a prescription for senna beside their beds! District nursing is certainly more than bathing elderly folk whose relatives think they need a wash," I continued.

"My aul grandda never had a bath in his life, but he was perfectly clean. I canna understand why folk are so desperate for their grannies to be bathed. Naebody has died for want of a bath but plenty hae died haeing ane!" Muriel replied.

"I don't know how often we hear of folk falling in the bath, or being stuck there all night," I agreed. "Seventy-five per cent of accidents at home happen in the bathroom."

Florence Nightingale had washed the soldiers in Scutari, even though their drinking water was so contaminated they succumbed to dysentery and typhoid fever, rather than dirt, so nurses continue to wash their patients enthusiastically.

A lady Muriel and Evelyn visited lived in total squalor.

"Mrs Steele hasna' seen a bar of soap in years. We'll hae to get the environmental health people in to clean her flat. You and me Evelyn will tak her to the hospital and delouse her," Muriel explained.

"OK. We'll take a crown car though, and cover the seats with polythene. There's no way we're taking her in either of our cars. We'd itch forever afterwards," Evelyn said.

The shock of it all was too great, and Mrs Steele died a week later.

"I feel really guilty aboot that wifie. If we hadna come and bothered her she'd maybe still be here today," Muriel said.

"She'll be looking down at us from the happy land, all sparkling clean inside and out," Evelyn replied.

"I'm glad I missed out on that one!" said Gail. "But come on OBE, it's time to visit Mrs Poli, how's your Italian today?"

Mrs Poli lived with her two sons, Alfredo and Giovanni. She was depressed, but Evelyn had her singing Italian, Gaelic and Scottish songs in the bath.

Evelyn tried to teach us some Gaelic too.

"Seo," she would say, handing me the soap. "That means 'here,' and you must say 'tapadach leat', which means 'thank you'." I repeated it after her, but in the heat of the moment I could never pronounce the words properly.

"Your Gaelic is as bad as your driving, Margaret," Evelyn said with mock despair.

"The problem with old Mrs Poli is the parrot," Gail said. "They let it out to fly about the room. Evelyn hates the sudden way it swoops down beside you."

"I always go there early," Evelyn said. "The parrot's never up before ten o'clock."

"Mrs Poli usually offers me a sweet from the dish beside her chair," Gail continued. "I had a tickly dry throat the other day, so I took a sweetie without her asking me first and that blooming bird shouted out, 'Naughty, naughty!' "

One day I happened to meet Giovanni on the bus going into town. He had bad news for me.

"The parrot's dead."

"Oh dear," I replied. "Your mother will be sad about that."

"Yes," he sighed. "But it's worse for me, the parrot passed away in my hands. I'm seeing my counsellor today. He's helping me come to terms with my loss."

Giovanni died soon afterwards, in the cafeteria at the hospital. He had developed cancer and was in hospital for treatment. He visited the cafe with his brother one day and died of a heart attack.

Patients with multiple sclerosis sometimes needed a great deal of nursing care to meet the complexities of their disabilities. We nursed a lady who became totally helpless. Her name was Jessie. She lived alone and relied on nurses and home helps to look after her.

"I can only move my richt hand a bittie, and I'm left handed," Jessie told us sadly.

"Jessie's a fine wifie, but she's gey thrawn," Muriel said in despair.

"She winna go to bed because the spasms get worse, so she sits in her wheelchair a' nicht. Her legs are really swollen."

"Weel, quines," Jessie told Muriel and Gail one day. " I've ordered a reclining chair, so I'll be able to put my feet up. It'll be like lying doon in my bed."

"Aye, but you're still nae getting off your bum," Muriel objected. "So you're still at risk of pressure sores."

"I'm nae going to my bed. I canna move and when the spasms start I'm so sair I canna thole it," Jessie said with determination. "Besides I canna hae a fag if I'm lying doon."

When the reclining chair came, Jessie had to be lifted out of it into a wheel chair, taken through to her bed to be washed, and given the nursing care she needed. Then she was lifted back into her wheelchair, and then back into the reclining chair. All this was accompanied by cries because lifting her brought on the spasms. She became very distressed when a hoist was suggested to save the nurses' backs from injury as well as to make it easier on herself.

"We'll hae to bring in a hoist, Jessie. The managers are aye on aboot safety. I'll get into trouble if we dinna hae ane in the hoose," Muriel pleaded.

"Weel, you can bring it in, but I'm nae ginging into it for ony manager," Jessie said with her usual spirit.

One day Jessie announced she was having a party to celebrate her seventieth birthday.

"You quines are a' invited, and I'm asking a' my freends I eesed tae ken at the Bingo and the disabled swimming. I fairly miss getting oot tae a' those things. Mind I'm nae wanting ony presents, but you can gie a contribution towards buying things for the common room here wha I bide. I'm asking a' the folkies here an a'. We'll hae oor party in the common room, and it'll be a fine nicht for you a' tae min' on faur when I'm nae langer here."

We had a great night with dancing and singing as well as heaps of food and drink.

Jessie had a good singing voice and joined in all the songs with gusto.

"I canna get up tae dance but I can still sing a bittie. Are you haeing a fine time quines?" she asked us. She could tell that we were indeed enjoying it all as much as she was.

"Jessie, that was a really good night out, thank you so much," Gail said as we left at the end of the evening. We were all pleased to see Jessie so happy.

"It's fine to see oor Jessie haeing a guid time instead o' greeting because she disna wants us to lift her oot o' her chair," Muriel remarked. "This has been better than ony medicine the doctor could gie her. She'll hae plenty tae speak aboot wi' a' the nurses for the next whilie."

Jessie liked all the nurses, the weekend ones, the evening ones and the night sisters who visited if she called them out in an emergency.

"All the quines are richt guid," she'd say.

There was a male nurse who worked at the weekends. Jessie liked him too.

"That's a fine loon. He kens fit wey tae lift me"

Jessie tried all sorts of alternative therapies to help herself. She enjoyed Shiatsu and reflexology.

"Maybe you should try cannabis," I suggested half jokingly. "It's supposed to help the spasms. But you mustn't tell anyone it was my idea."

"Na, na, I'm nae for that. I ken the spasms are bad and nae drugs are ony eese, but I dinna want tae be a junkie. I'll stick to my fags. The hoast they gie me fairly helps the bowels!"

Jessie's home help, and the lady who was the cleaner in the sheltered housing complex where she lived were very good to her. They would pop in at weekends with shopping or just to check up on her and keep her company. They were friends as well as paid helpers.

As her illness progressed, night nurses sat with her all night because she was terrified to go to hospital and refused to consider the idea. She died peacefully at home, so her wish was realised.

We were all a bit down after Jessie died.

"Let's go horse riding one evening," Muriel suggested. "Mind we went pony trekking up at Balmoral last year?"

"I didn't manage to go with you that time," I said. "But you've got the photo of yourself riding the Queen's horse on your desk to prove you were there. I'd come with you this time, but I can't ride. The last time I was on a horse was donkey's years ago." I told her about the experience I'd had as a new student nurse.

"If I'm on a horse that bolts again, I'll disappear off into the sunset. When the patients ask 'where's the nurse?' you can say I was last seen galloping in the direction of Clachnaben."

"You needna' worry. I keep my horse at a riding stables and there will be instructors to lead you if you need help," Muriel said reassuringly.

By now Muriel had bought a horse with the help and advice of Linda who was an experienced horsewoman.

"Well, I've heard you and Linda talk about your horse so much, I'll give it a go." I decided.

"I'll come as well," Gail said.

"I canna come," Sheila put in.

"Can you nae get a baby sitter, Sheila?" Muriel asked. "I could mak it a different time to suit you."

"You'll hae to wait nine months then," Sheila said with a smile.

"That's surely the hot seat where you two sit," Gail joked. "That's Linda back after her second baby, and now it's you again, Sheila."

We had an evening of riding amongst the rolling Deeside hills. A riding instructor led me on my horse and so I didn't have any worries about getting the animal to obey me.

"I've got something to tell you all," Evelyn announced one day. "I'm retiring in September."

We all knew that Evelyn was thinking about retiring, but we also all knew how much she would be missed by us and by all her patients.

We had a big party for her, and she left showered with gifts from so many people, patients and colleagues alike.

"I don't know how the Aberdonians get a reputation for meanness, Margaret," Evelyn said. "I'm totally overwhelmed with such generosity."

"I know. They're not so outgoing as the Glasgow folk, but they're good hearted when you get to know them. Mind you, we've come across some beauties in our day haven't we?" I said. "Remember that old horror, Miss Robertson, and poor old Snuffy Ivy? And what about that Mrs Steele you and Muriel deloused and then she died?"

"And there was the day I thought I saw a ghost, when Mrs Watt was suspended in mid air. And what about me and the parrot, and you with all your brushes with the law, Margaret? I think it would be good to write a book about all the folk we've looked after, and all the changes you and I have seen over the years," Evelyn said.

"That's what I said to Katie once," I remembered. "But we're nurses, not writers. Who knows, maybe once I'm retired I'll manage to put all these things down on paper."

And so I have.

Layout: Stephen M.L. Young
                 latouveilhe@mac.com

Font: Adobe Garamond (11pt)

Copies of this book can be ordered via the Internet:

                 www.librario.com

or from:

                 Librario Publishing Ltd
                 Brough House
                 Milton Brodie
                 Kinloss
                 Moray IV36 2UA
                 Tel /Fax No 01343 850 617